D0759462

Alternative Immunoassays

Alternative Immunoassays

Edited by

W. P. Collins
Professor of Reproductive Biochemistry and
Director of Diagnostics Research Unit,
Department of Obstetrics and Gynaecology,
King's College School of Medicine and Dentistry,
Denmark Hill, London, UK

A Wiley Medical Publication

JOHN WILEY & SONS
Chichester · New York · Brisbane · Toronto · Singapore

Library of Congress Cataloging in Publication Data:
Main entry under title:

Alternative immunoassays.

(A Wiley medical publication)
Includes index.
1. Immunoassay. 2. Biomolecules—Analysis.
I. Collins, W. P. II. Series. [DNLM: 1. Immunoassay.
2. Immunoassay—methods. QW 570 A 466]
OP519.9.I42A44   1985   616.07'56   84-26923
ISBN 0 471 90669 7

British Library Cataloguing in Publication Data:

Alternative immunoassays.—(A
Wiley medical publication)
1. Immunoassay
I. Collins, W.P.
616.07'56   RB46.5

ISBN 0 471 90669 7

Typeset by Photo·graphics Ltd., Honiton
Printed and Bound in Great Britain

List of contributors

S. R. Abbott, Boots–Celltech Diagnostics Ltd, Slough, UK

T. S. Baker, Boots–Celltech Diagnostics Ltd, Slough, UK

G. J. R. Barnard, Diagnostics Research Unit, Department of Obstetrics and Gynaecology, King's College School of Medicine and Dentistry, London, UK

D. E. Bidwell, Department of Clinical Tropical Medicine, London School of Hygiene and Tropical Medicine, London, UK

J. De Boever, Department of Obstetrics and Gynaecology, Academic Hospital, Gent, Belgium

A. K. Campbell, Department of Medical Biochemistry, Welsh National School of Medicine, Cardiff, UK

W. P. Collins, Diagnostics Research Unit, Department of Obstetrics and Gynaecology, King's College School of Medicine and Dentistry, London, UK

S. G. Daniel, Boots–Celltech Diagnostics Ltd, Slough, UK

R. P. Ekins, Department of Molecular Endocrinology, The Middlesex Hospital Medical School, London, UK

T. C. J. Gribnau, Diagnostic Research Laboratories, Organon International BV, Oss, The Netherlands

P. Halonen, Department of Virology, University of Turku, Turku, Finland

H. van Hell, Diagnostic Research Laboratories, Organon International BV, Oss, The Netherlands

I. Hemmilä, Wallac Biochemical Laboratory, Turku, Finland

S. L. Jeffcoate, Department of Biochemical Endocrinology, Chelsea Hospital for Women, London, UK

J. B. Kim, Diagnostics Research Unit, Department of Obstetrics and Gynaecology, King's College School of Medicine and Dentistry, London, UK

F.Kohen, Department of Hormone Research, The Weitzmann Institute of Science, Rehovot, Israel

J. Landon, Department of Chemical Pathology, St Bartholomew's Hospital, London, UK

J. H. W. Leuvering, Diagnostic Research Laboratories, Organon International BV, Oss, The Netherlands

T. Lovgren, Wallac Biochemical Laboratory, Turku, Finland

V. Marks, Division of Clinical Biochemistry, University of Surrey, Guildford, UK

A. Patel, Department of Medical Biochemistry, Welsh National School of Medicine, Cardiff, UK

M. Pazzagli, Institute of Endocrinology, University of Florence, Italy

K. Pettersson, Wallac Biochemical Laboratory, Turku, Finland

P. A. Roberts, Department of Medical Biochemistry, Welsh National School of Medicine, Cardiff, UK

M. Serio, Institute of Endocrinology, University of Florence, Italy

K. Siddle, Department of Clinical Biochemistry, University of Cambridge, Addenbrooke's Hospital, Cambridge, UK

A. M. Sidki, Department of Chemical Pathology, St Bartholomew's Hospital, London, UK

E. Soini, Wallac Oy, Turku, Finland

D. Vandekerckhove, Department of Obstetrics and Gynaecology, Academic Hospital, Gent, Belgium

A. Voller, Immunodiagnostics Unit, Nuffield Laboratories of Comparative Medicine, Institute of Zoology, The Zoological Society of London, UK

J. L. Williams, Diagnostics Research Unit, Department of Obstetrics and Gynaecology, King's College School of Medicine and Dentistry, London, UK

J. F. Wright, Boots–Celltech Diagnostics Ltd, Slough, UK

Contents

Preface

Immunoassays with radioactive and non-isotopic tracers were developed at almost the same time approximately 25 years ago. It became apparent, however, that radioimmunoassay was the most appropriate of these procedures for measuring most kinds of analyte with good sensitivity, specificity and precision. There are three main, non-commerical reasons for the recent revival of interest in alternative immunoassays. The first is the advent of monoclonal antibodies, the second is the trend towards the development of simple extra-laboratory tests, and the third is the application of more efficient and safer forms of luminescence to achieve higher sensitivity. A symposium was held at the Institute of Psychiatry, University of London, during November 1983 to report and evaluate current alternative immunoassays, and to predict future trends and applications. The proceedings were reported in *Medical Laboratory World*, January 1984, pp.37–41, and a succinct review of immunoassay developments with a selected bibliography appeared in the *Bibliography of Reproduction* **44** (2), 1984, pp.A1–A8. The chapters for this book were written during January to July 1984 and are a more detailed, updated, reflection on topics covered at the meeting. More recently, a non-isotopic immunometric assay has been published for the measurement of haptens (*Clin. Chem.* **30**, 1984, pp.1494–1498), and an evanescent wave immunoassay has been promulgated for the rapid measurement of analytes – based on reaction rates, with or without the use of a label (*Clin. Chem.* **30**, 1984, pp.1533–1538).

I predict that the development of immunometric assays for the measurement of both proteins and haptens will continue to fulfil the theoretical advantages, and even the limitations may be exploited. The choice of label will depend upon the sensitivity required, the location of the test, and the prejudice of the consumer. It is probable that more novel reagents will be produced by genetic manipulation, and that the introduction of alternative technologies will be gradual. It is hoped that the information contained in this book will be of interest to research workers, and will help managers of diagnostic services to plan their future requirements.

December 1984   W. P. COLLINS

Nomenclature

To date, there is no definitive method for the classification and description of diagnostic tests which involve the binding of antigens to antibodies. A widely used approach which covers most situations is based upon whether or not the concentration of antibody binding sites is limited. Accordingly, the methods may be classified as competitive binding, limited reagent immunoassays, or non-competitive, excess reagent immunometric assays. Secondary, descriptive criteria involve the type of label (e.g. radioimmunoassay or immunoradiometric assay), and the method of detection if it is not apparent (e.g. enzyme fluoroimmunoassay or immunoenzymofluorometric assay). A third factor which is often described is the type of solid phase (e.g. sol particle immunoassay), which may also be the label. Many confusing situations may arise. For example, a labelled second antibody may be used in excess to monitor a competitive binding immunoassay, and if the free fraction is measured in an excess reagent method the procedure may also be considered to be competitive. In addition, an antibody may be the analyte, and the antigen or antibody may be linked to a solid phase. In addition, the methods may be subdivided into those which involve a physical separation of the assay mixture before the end point is determined (i.e. the heterogeneous or separation assays), or those where a measurement is taken in the presence of all reactants (i.e. the homogeneous or non-separation assays). In this book the classification of assays and the associated terminology reflects the preferences of the individual authors.

CHAPTER 1

Uses of immunoassay

V. Marks
Division of Clinical Biochemistry,
University of Surrey, Guildford, Surrey GU2 5XH, UK

1. INTRODUCTION

Antibodies have been used as diagnostic reagents, in one form or another, for more than half a century, but immunoassay as we understand it today began with the application by Yalow and Berson, in 1959, of anti-insulin antibodies to the measurement of the hormone in plasma. For the next 10 years or so immunoassay was used almost exclusively by biomedical investigators for measuring polypeptide hormones in plasma and other biological fluids. Much of the developmental work on immunoassay during this period was concerned with improving labelling techniques, methods of separating bound and free label, and antibody production (Abraham, 1977). Workers in other industries, and practitioners of disciplines other than endocrinology within biomedical research, were slow to recognize the enormous potential of immunoassay for helping to solve their analytical problems. The first major breakthrough came with the rediscovery of Landsteiner's (1945) work on antibody production against low molecular weight haptens and the realization that immunoassay could be applied to the measurement of drugs in biological fluids, often without the necessity of performing elaborate clean-up procedures. During the 1970s, and particularly during the latter half of the decade, there was an explosive growth in the application of immunoassay to other biomedical disciplines as well as to industries which had hitherto had little or no contact with immunology.

1

2. CLINICAL PRACTICE

Technical problems, mostly due to difficulties in obtaining reagents, ensured that the use of immunoassay was confined largely to research groups during the first 10 years following its discovery. The commercial introduction of pre-packed reagents (kits), first for the measurement of insulin, but subsequently for other polypeptide hormones, enabled any well equipped hospital laboratory to perform immunoassays, provided that appropriate instrumentation was available. The earliest commercial reagents all relied upon the use of radioisotopic labels—either ^{125}I or ^{3}H—and therefore demanded access to gamma and/or liquid scintillation counters, neither of which had previously been considered standard clinical laboratory equipment. The introduction of enzyme labels (Pal, 1978), particularly when incorporated into so-called homogeneous (i.e. non-separation) techniques, with their requirement for nothing more elaborate than a spectrophotometer for measurement, led to a rapid expansion of immunoassay in clinical laboratories throughout the developed world. Today there must be very few laboratories, serving hospitals with over 500 beds, that do not have facilities for performing at least some immunoassays for diagnostic and monitoring purposes.

The range of tests performed in clinical laboratories spread rapidly following the introduction of pre-packed reagents, especially when kits using other than radioactive labels became available. The main emphasis remains in endocrinology, which demands the exquisite sensitivity, specificity and ability for performance on unextracted samples that immunoassay alone can offer. Nowadays, however, the immunoassay repertoire includes not only the polypeptide hormones, but also the various steroid hormones and amino acid derivatives—notably thyroxine and triiodothyronine. Other divisions of the clinical laboratory that make extensive use of immunoassay include those involved in monitoring the management of infertility and fetal well-being, the detection of proteinopathies, toxicology and, above all, therapeutic drug monitoring (Richens and Marks, 1981). The ability to simplify the analytical processes to such an extent that they can be performed rapidly with minimum effort at the patient's bedside, or in the outpatient clinic, has made immunoassay the method of choice.

Although the vast majority of immunoassays are still performed on human blood plasma (or serum), an increasingly large number are being undertaken on other biological fluids, notably urine, saliva, cerebrospinal and synovial fluids, milk and tissue extracts. Skin swabs have been analysed by immunoassay for the detection of drug abuse and/or explosives, and blood spots prepared in the home by health visitors or by patients themselves are being used increasingly for screening or monitoring of disease.

Immunoassay currently remains largely the prerogative of clinical biochemistry within laboratory medicine but this situation is unlikely to continue for much longer (Voller *et al.*, 1981). Already the microbiologists are recognizing its merits as a means of identifying and quantitating viruses, certain bacteria and their toxic products, antibodies and antibiotics. Immunohistology (Polak and Van Noorden, 1983) has developed apace since it was first used to identify and localize autoimmune disease. In haematology, immunoassay has been adapted to the investigation of disorders of coagulation and fibrinolysis.

3. VETERINARY MEDICINE, HORTICULTURE AND AGRICULTURE

The application of immunoassay techniques to the solution of problems arising in veterinary practice was at first confined, as in medicine, to research, but the increasing availability of various kits has brought the technique within the scope of many practitioners (Morris and Bolton, 1984). The most common application remains the early detection of pregnancy, but increasingly immunoassay is being applied to the prediction and confirmation of ovulation, the investigation of metabolic disorders, the detection of toxins in milk and/or flesh, and the detection of infectious diseases. In horse racing, as in human sport, immunoassay has become the screening method of choice for detecting drug abuse prior to more specific identification by gas chromatography—mass spectrometry (GC-MS). Agriculturalists have latterly come to recognize the potential value of immunoassay for detecting and quantifying toxins in plants and animals, but above all for recognizing real or impending viral and other infections of plants and animals before they have had a chance to wreak economic havoc.

4. FOOD INDUSTRY

The food industry has always depended heavily upon analytical technology, but the benefits to be gained from the greater use of immunoassays have only recently begun to be appreciated (Morris and Clifford, 1984). Undoubtedly the greatest stumbling block to its more rapid application in the food industry has been the shortage of suitable reagents, which have not, as in the biomedical field, had the advantage of being developed, in the first instance, as a spin-off of fundamental research sponsored and paid for by government agencies and/or medical charities. Now that the enormous potential for immunoassay in the food industry has been recognized, however, the entry of enterprising manufacturers into the market can be expected. In the future, immunoassay may be used for many analyses that are currently being undertaken with more tedious, and hence more expensive, procedures. The measurement of the vitamin content of food, various additives—including colourants—as well as the detection and quantitation of specific toxins and pesticide residues are examples of the uses to which immunoassay can be put.

An application for which the need has been recognized, but the means have not yet materialized, is the adulteration (or accidental contamination) of one kind of footstuff by another, e.g. the illicit addition of vegetable to animal protein in pre-packed food, or the passing-off of inferior meats (e.g. kangaroo or donkey) as beef or lamb.

5. ENVIRONMENTAL HEALTH

Increasing awareness of the possible role of toxic materials in the environment in the genesis of diverse diseases has placed greater reliance upon sensitive analytical procedures than ever before. The application of immunoassay to this problem is comparatively recent, but the past few years have seen its employment for the detection of antibiotic, pesticide, herbicide, detergent and other real or potentially toxic residues in the atmosphere, piped and well waters, and vegetation. Immunoassays have also been used to detect xenobiotics in the flesh (and, where relevant, eggs) of wild birds, fish and other animals as evidence of past or continuing environmental pollution.

6. FORENSIC SCIENCE

The exquisite sensitivity coupled with the remarkable (group) specificity of immunoassay led to its relatively early application to the detection of drug abuse both for clinical and forensic purposes. Frequently the small size of the sample, e.g. a blood or saliva spot, or a semen stain, may dictate the use of methods with analytical sensitivity and specificity possessed by no other technique than immunoassay; this advantage is even more important when the substance being sought is a protein which is identified by nothing more than its immunological characteristics, (e.g. blood group substances and tissue antigens). It is in these applications that monoclonal antibodies have established their superiority as analytical and identification reagents.

Though radioimmunoassay remains the most popular method of performing immunoassay in biomedical research and clinical work—mainly because it was firmly established before equally effective alternative methods became available—this is not so in other industries, where enzyme, fluorescent or chemiluminescent techniques, in one or more of their diverse forms, have a large share of the rapidly growing market. Automated equipment suitable for use with these methods is still in its infancy, but the time is not far off when much of the routine analytical work currently performed in many industries by classical chemical techniques will be undertaken by immunoassay. The impending introduction of solid phase immunoelectrodes (biosensors) with exquisite sensitivity and unimaginably short response times will permit continuous downstream monitoring in manufacturing industries and others, e.g. the supply of fresh water and the disposal of sewage.

REFERENCES

Abraham, G.E. (1977). *Handbook of Radioimmunoassay*. Marcel Dekker, New York.

Landsteiner, K. (1945). *Specificity of Serological Reactions*, Charles C. Thomas, Springfield, Ill.

Morris, B.A., and Bolton, A.E. (1985). *Immunoassays in Veterinary Practice*, Ellis Horwood, Chichester, in press.

Morris, B.A., and Clifford, M.N. (1985). *Immunoassays in Food Analysis*, Elsevier Applied Science, London, in press.

Pal, S.B. (1978). *Enzyme Labelled Immunoassay of Hormones and Drugs*, Walter de Gruyter, Berlin.

Polak, J.M., and Van Noorden, S. (1983). *Immunocytochemistry: Practical Applications in Pathology and Biology*, John Wright, Bristol.

Richens, A., and Marks, V. (1981). *Therapeutic Drug Monitoring*, Churchill Livingstone, Edinburgh.

Voller, A., Bartlett, A., and Bidwell, D. (1981). *Immunoassays for the 80s*, MTP, Lancaster.

Alternative Immunoassays
Edited by W. P. Collins
© 1985 John Wiley & Sons Ltd

CHAPTER 2

Advantages and limitations of traditional technology

S. L. JEFFCOATE

Department of Biochemical Endocrinology,
Chelsea Hospital for Women,
Dovehouse Street,
London SW3 6LJ, UK

1. INTRODUCTION

The few modest contributions that I made to immunoassay technology were over a decade ago and this chapter is written by a current consumer of such technology rather than a creator. My department has multiple analytical functions encompassing clinical, research and postgraduate teaching activities in the field of reproductive endocrinology. Over 30 000 analyses are carried out per year of over 15 different analytes including both peptide and steroid hormones measured mainly in samples from human subjects, though also from rodents, and mainly blood serum or plasma, though also other body fluids such as urine and saliva. These analytes are present in picomolar or nanomolar concentrations and to this analytical constraint is added the need to maintain a clinical service with reliable turn-around and quality of results.

I have given this background in some detail since it inevitably influences my judgement of immunoassay methods—both 'traditional' and 'alternative'. Consequently the comments and decisions that I make as the manager of such an analytical service may not be applicable to, or representative of, other fields where the analytical requirements are quite different (e.g. toxicology in the food industry; protozoal antigens in Africa; pharmacology).

2. ALTERNATIVE TO WHAT?

The methods used in our laboratory are highly refined versions of what some people would disparagingly call 'first generation' immunoassay technology. We use liquid-phase incubation with polyclonal antibodies and radioactive labels. The separation of free and antibody-bound fractions is achieved by simple precipitation (e.g. with second antibody) or adsorption (e.g. with charcoal) methodology. We use work-simplified semi-automated procedures, but eschew automated pipetting, dispensing and/or incubation systems as being inappropriate for our particular needs. Our methods are cheap, rugged and applicable to a wide variety of analytes. Quality control and trouble-shooting procedures are well established and staff training and laboratory equipment are geared to these methods (Jeffcoate, 1981).

Thus, we ask ourselves, why change? At a time of economic constraint, investment in new equipment is difficult and any new laboratory procedure may involve re-training in all aspects of laboratory practice. Immunoassay, as we practise it, has represented a 'quantum leap' in analytical biochemistry in the past 20 years (equivalent to the self-loading compared to the flint-lock rifle, or the pocket calculator compared to the slide-rule) and it will require an equivalent leap to persuade us to change now. Many of the current alternative technologies, however, do offer potential advantages that ought to be considered, and I would like to discuss the relationship between these possible improvements, and the objectives of our analytic service.

3. POSSIBLE ADVANTAGES OF ALTERNATIVE TECHNOLOGIES

The many possible advantages (analytical, clinical and practical) of new methodologies overlap, and indeed are interdependent. Analytical benefits would result if the sources of error leading respectively to: (i) within-batch imprecision; (ii) between-batch variability, and (iii) method-associated bias (inaccuracy) could be minimized. In general within-batch imprecision values of 3–5% coefficient of variation, over about two orders of magnitude of analyte concentration, are achievable with conventional immunoassay methods. Important benefits could accrue if the working range could be extended downwards to smaller analyte concentrations (increased sensitivity) and/or broadened to cover more than two orders of magnitude. In general this would increase the useful applications of the assay systems. In the endocrine field, for example, this could allow measurement of low levels of human thyrotropin (hTSH) not possible with limited reagent, competitive binding methods and the precise measurement of high levels after a stimula-tion test without the necessity for prior sample dilution (see Chapters 3 and 5 of this volume). Of the analytical benefits, an increase in assay ruggedness, with an improvement of between-batch reproducibility, would be a major advantage leading to more reliable assays, a more efficient clinical service and reduced costs. A reduction of method bias does not necessarily follow from technical advances (in fact, the opposite may occur).

Improved comparability of potency estimates between centres, whether through the use of common reagents and protocols or otherwise, has important economic and scientific advantages. Careful standardization and multicentre collaborative studies are required to achieve this objective. At the practical level, technical advances can also lead to simpler, faster and cheaper methods, which may in turn expand the clinical applications of the assays, e.g. to new body fluids, to subfractions of analytes, and to the development of bedside tests.

In the following sections I will examine some of the currently proposed alternatives and indicate my personal view of their real or potential value.

4. ALTERNATIVE LABELS

Three types of labelling are applicable: those in which the ligand is labelled (immunoassays); those in which the binding reagent or ligate is labelled (immunometric assays); and those in which the physicochemical changes associated with antibody binding can be observed without an additional label (unlabelled assays). In the unlabelled assays the absence of a tracer means that there is one less reagent to assess and control, but the methods are only applicable to concentrations of analyte many orders of magnitude higher than those encountered in most situations. Labelled ligand assays require appropriate supplies of purified materials. Labelled ligate assays offer theoretical advantages and are generally used in solid-phase or sandwich assay systems (see Chapters 3, 5, 9, 12 and 13 of this volume).

The following labels are widely used as alternatives to radionuclides: (i) enzymes (or their substrates or cofactors), and (ii) luminescent compounds (either fluorescent or chemiluminescent). These labels in turn govern the nomenclature of the assays, depending on whether the ligand (enzymoimmunoassay, fluoroimmunoassay or chemiluminoimmunoassay) or ligate (immunoenzymometric, immunofluorometric, immunochemiluminometric assays) is labelled. The advantages of non-isotopic methods will be detailed elsewhere in this volume, but essentially relate to the hazards of handling radioactivity (often small, however, in comparison to other laboratory hazards) and the longer shelf-life of non-isotopic tracers.

When used as an end-point signal in immunoassay, radioactivity has one principal advantage and one major disadvantage. With appropriate equipment, counting strategies and conventional amounts of radionuclide, the imprecision due to counting error is extremely small (coefficients of variation in the range 0.1–1.0%), and the values are effectively negligible in comparison with other experimental errors in the system. Alternative tracers with their appropriate detection systems have to match this precision in those analyses for which it is required. There are, of course, semi-quantitative or all-or-none (yes/no) analyses where precision in the signal measurement is less important and for which the high precision of radioactive counting is not required. The major drawback to the use of radionuclides is the waste of signal. To take an example:^{125}I, with a half-life of 60 days, emits only 1/100 000th of its potential within 1 min and 99.999% of the radioactivity is not used (and indeed becomes a disposal problem). Tracers which emit all of their signal are thus potentially capable of producing assays with considerably lower detection points.

5. ALTERNATIVE PROCEDURES

A very large variety of alternative procedures has been explored in recent years (e.g. solid-phase assays, non-separation assays, sandwich assays) including many systems introduced (and patented) by commercial companies and marketed under strange acronyms (e.g. CELIA, LIDIA, SPIA, CLASP). The objectives behind these developments include improvements in ruggedness, simplicity, throughput, cheapness or the need to evade patents. Many of these variations, with their corresponding advantages and disadvantages, will be discussed in the pages that follow, and the only general comment worth making is a repetition of an earlier one: the decision whether an alternative immunoassay procedure should replace a traditional one rests with the user and he/she should decide having considered whether the changes in analytical quality (sensitivity, bias, precision and ruggedness), practicality (cost, ease of use, speed) and/or clinical applications are, on balance, appropriate for his/her particular analytical needs.

My particular requirements in a specialized endocrine laboratory associated with a postgraduate teaching hospital in a European capital city are clearly different from those of an epidemiologist measuring the prevalence of protozoal antigen-positive subjects in Brazilian rain forests and in general terms the immunoassay procedures *per se* represent only a small fraction of the time, costs and sources of error involved in providing an effective and efficient analytical service. Other factors such as sample collection, transport, reception and storage, and the preparation, storage, transport and, above, all, interpretation of the report form, are areas where improvements are more necessary in my field of interest than in the analytical process itself.

6. ALTERNATIVE BODY FLUIDS

The dependence on blood sampling for most current immunoassays (in endocrinology at least) has the drawback that it requires a trained phlebotomist and is uncomfortable for the patient: this limitation is especially apparent if serial measurements are needed to monitor dynamic physiological or pathological situations. So-called non-invasive sampling, of urine or saliva for example, would thus be superior provided that these fluids gave an adequate reflection of the pathophysiological parameters under investigation and provided that analytical quality was appropriate.

In this context, saliva is increasingly advocated as an alternative fluid to blood plasma for assays (Read *et al.*, 1984). From the practical viewpoint it is clearly easier to obtain, and subjects can collect serial samples without attendance at hospital. The specimens may even be stored at home until a series is complete. We now have considerable experience of collecting and assaying such samples, including the organization of world-wide, multicentre trials. The major practical difficulty appears to lie in the variable—and often undesirable—eating and smoking habits and standards of oral hygiene between individual subjects and racial and national groups. This situation can make the samples unpleasant—even repulsive—for the laboratory staff to handle.

Another suggested advantage of salivary steroid assays is that saliva is an ultrafiltrate of plasma, and only the free (non-protein-bound) and biologically available fraction is present: thus salivary steroid levels reflect the biologically active fraction. Unfortunately this view is based on two erroneous suppositions. First, saliva is not a simple ultrafiltrate and steroids are excreted in it via three different routes: (i) by ultrafiltration through the gap junctions; (ii) by transport through the cell; and (iii) by contamination from blood or gingival fluid. Transport through the cell may involve metabolism of the steroid and contamination will include all plasma fractions. The other major misconception is concerned with the bio-availability of protein-bound steroids in plasma. It is now clear that albumin binding has only a minimal effect on tissue availability because dissociation of steroids from it is rapid compared with the capillary transit time. In some situations even steroids bound to high affinity binding globulins can be available for tissue uptake. Thus whilst salivary steroid concentrations reflect plasma levels they are much lower (1–2%) and their measurement is not necessarily an improvement on plasma assays on either practical or theoretical grounds.

7. WHY ALTERNATIVE IMMUNOASSAYS MAY REMAIN ALTERNATIVES

In conclusion, it seems to me that the currently available and developing alternatives to traditional immunoassay methods do not contribute a sufficiently major improvement to warrant the effort and expense involved in making the change. It will require a 'quantum leap' equivalent to that which radioimmunoassay represented in the 1960s to bring about the conditions where a change is worthwhile. In addition to necessitating the re-training of personnel and the purchase of new equipment, changes in methodology are associated with (perhaps temporary) uncertainties about quality control, sources of error, trouble-shooting and interpretation of results. One particular aspect of the doubts that I have is that no single alternative (e.g. chemiluminescence assays) is yet emerging as a clear leader. We do not wish to have multiple different types of methodology in one department, so until one alternative is shown to be superior we shall wait.

A final difficulty with the widespread acceptance of alternative technologies, in the UK at least, is that most developments are taking place in commercial companies with an inevitable competitive and defensive approach to patenting, increased expense and worst of all the resultant dependence of the consumer on the supply of particular reagents and, often, machines. For all these reasons, whilst I remain openminded about the future, my laboratory will be staying with traditional immunoassays for the time being.

REFERENCES

Jeffcoate, S.L. (1981). *Efficiency and Effectiveness in the Endocrine Laboratory*, Academic Press, London.

Read, G.F., Riad-Fahmy, D., Walker, R.F., and Griffiths, K. (1984). *Immunoassays of steroids in Saliva (Proceedings of the Ninth Tenovus Workshop)*, Alpha Omega Publishing, Cardiff.

Alternative Immunoassays
Edited by W. P. Collins
© 1985 John Wiley & Sons Ltd

CHAPTER 3

Properties and applications of monoclonal antibodies

K. SIDDLE

Department of Clinical Biochemistry, University of Cambridge,
Addenbrooke's Hospital,
Hills Road,
Cambridge CB2 2QR, UK

1. INTRODUCTION

Monoclonal antibodies have in recent years made an enormous impact on many areas of biomedical research, but have not yet become widely used in diagnostic immunoassays. To some extent this reflects the considerable effort which must be put into obtaining antibodies suitable for use in methods which must satisfy demanding standards of sensitivity and specificity. There has also been some tendency to look on monoclonal antibodies merely as alternatives to polyclonal antisera for use in existing competitive radioimmunoassay techniques. When good polyclonal antisera are available in sufficient quantity, it has not seemed worthwhile to go to the trouble of obtaining monoclonal antibodies as simple replacements. Moreover, although monoclonality is an undoubted benefit, in terms of reproducibility and availability of antibody, it does not in itself ensure a better reagent than polyclonal serum, because of the critical importance of affinity and specificity in determining assay performance. Thus, it should not be expected that a first small set of monoclonal antibodies will immediately prove superior to tried and tested antisera, which are possibly the selected product of years of immunization of many animals in several laboratories. It will often be necessary to produce and characterize a large number of monoclonal antibodies for a given antigen, in order to identify a few of exceptional properties, and to consider various different ways of making use of these in diagnostic methods.

13

Table 1. Some properties of monoclonal antibodies

Advantages over polyclonal antisera

1. Indefinite supply of antibody with constant characteristics
2. Monospecific antibody obtained from impure immunogen
3. Affinity and fine specificity are defined and may be selected to suit application
4. Availability of antibodies for multiple different and discrete epitopes on given antigen
5. Rapid equilibration in binding of antigen
6. Easy purification in large quantities by methods which do not damage immunoreactivity
7. Clean reagents giving low non-specific binding and background
8. Often do not inhibit biological activity of antigen (e.g. enzymes)

Potential disadvantages

1. Low affinities predominate
2. Do not individually form precipitation lattices with most antigens
3. Do not always react with complement or protein A
4. May have unusual physical properties dependent on particular isotype or idiotype
5. Dependence on only a single epitope, which may not be representative of concentration or integrity of antigen as a whole (possibility of polymorphic or labile epitopes)

This chapter will attempt to underline the very real advantages which monoclonal antibodies possess as reagents for immunoassay (Table 1). This aim will involve a comparison not only of monoclonal and polyclonal antibodies, but also of different types of assay. Specific examples will be drawn largely from our own work, more general and widely referenced reviews being available elsewhere (Siddle, 1984, 1985). It will be seen that monoclonal antibodies are particularly powerful reagents when used in immunometric (labelled antibody) methods. Several companies have recently launched diagnostic kits offering assays of this type, and it is certain that these very rapid and sensitive methods will make an increasingly important contribution to diagnostic immunoassay.

2. PRODUCTION OF MONOCLONAL ANTIBODIES

The production of monoclonal antibodies is not technically difficult, but is relatively demanding in terms of time, effort and money. Detailed accounts of the principles and methods of production have been presented elsewhere (Galfre and Milstein, 1981; Bastin *et al.*, 1982), and only selected points will be considered here. In brief, spleen cells from immunized animals must be fused with myeloma cells growing in tissue culture, usually by using polyethylene glycol as the fusogen. The resulting suspension is distributed among a large number of small subcultures on tissue culture dishes. Cells are initially grown in a selective medium in which the unfused parental cells die, but hybrid cells survive and divide. Subcultures are screened to identify those cells (usually a small proportion of the total) which are making the specific antibody required. These cultures are not necessarily monoclonal at this stage, and one or more cloning steps are necessary to give stable, monoclonal cell lines. Subsequently the cell lines may be grown either in tissue culture, or as tumours in animals, in order to produce large quantities of antibody. Stable, antibody-producing hybrids are easily obtained only between cells of the same or closely related species, and the scope of the cell fusion technique is limited at present by the availability of suitable myeloma cell lines. Hence the antibodies currently produced are almost all of mouse or rat origin, although much effort is being directed towards the development of human hybridoma antibodies for use in man. As yet, it is not possible to immortalize the products of the immunoassayist's favourite animals such as rabbits and sheep, though the day may well come when this too will be feasible.

The production of monoclonal antibodies is a much more serious undertaking than simple immunization to obtain polyclonal antisera, and especially if work is carried out on the scale necessary to ensure (as far as this is ever possible) that some really good reagents will result. The technique ideally requires the individual attention of a small research team with specialist facilities and a considerable budget for consumables, and can therefore only be undertaken when real benefits are to be expected from the resulting antibodies. One consequence of these relative difficulties of production is that good monoclonal antibodies, even more than polyclonal antisera, are likely to be available only from a few specialist centres, and these are often commercial organizations rather than academic or hospital laboratories. The application of monoclonal antibodies may therefore lead of necessity, if not by design, to greater standardization of reagents and methodology, and to a more widespread use of assay kits rather than local 'in house' techniques.

2.1. Immunization

For those people who are intent on making their own monoclonal antibodies, the first requirement is to obtain a good preparation of immunogen, and to demonstrate a satisfactory immune response following its injection into mice or rats. The requirements for this stage of the proceedings are not markedly different from those for producing traditional polyclonal antisera. If anything, immunization is easier for monoclonal antibody production, because of the smaller amount of antigen needed per animal, and the less stringent requirements for its purity. The cloning and screening procedures used subsequently will ensure that only antibodies of chosen specificity are identified and processed, while other reactivities directed against impurities in the immunogen are discarded. It is worth noting that monoclonal antibodies, once obtained, are themselves, very powerful reagents for use in the affinity purification of the corresponding antigens (Secher and Burke, 1980; Dalchau and Fabre, 1982; Morgan et al., 1984; Jackson et al., 1984).

The outcome of a fusion experiment is dependent very largely on the success of the initial immunization. If the immunized animal is not producing a reasonable titre of antibody with required properties, then no amount of fusion of its spleen cells and cloning of hybrids can induce the formation of appropriate antibodies. Just as in the production of polyclonal antisera, there is therefore ample scope for injecting many animals, according to a variety of protocols, in order to identify the best responders for cell fusion. Such effort at this stage will certainly pay dividends, and help to avoid much fruitless work later.

Cell fusion is normally carried out only 4–5 days after a final intravenous booster immunization. This protocol gives rather little time for test bleeding and assessment of serum antibody response. We have found that the best prognostic index for a successful fusion is evidence of a rapid increase in titre following a final boost, rather than the absolute level of antibody at this stage.

Our preferred protocol is thus to identify good responders following a penultimate boost, rest these animals for some time to allow the serum antibody response to decline, and then to screen test bleeds before and after a final boost. On this basis, spleen cells from the best few animals from a larger group are chosen for fusion. Many different successful immunization protocols have been described in the literature (see, for example, Stähli et al., 1980), and this procedure is an aspect of the technique which still relies more on prejudice and anecdote than scientific study.

2.2. Cell fusion and screening

A variety of myeloma cell lines from mice and rats have been used successfully for cell fusions (Galfre and Milstein, 1981). It should be noted that some of these produce their own immunoglobulin chains, which become more or less randomly assembled with specific antibody chains of spleen cell origin in the products of the hybrid cell. Thus, truly homogeneous monoclonal antibodies are only obtained if non-producing myelomas are used for fusion. For many applications, the presence of a proportion of monovalent antibody, as arises if hybrids continue to produce light chains of myeloma origin, is not a problem. The generation of 'mixed' immunoglobulins has recently been turned to advantage, by using as fusion partners a hybrid myeloma making antibody of one specificity and spleen cells making a different antibody. The resulting 'second generation' hybrids produce a complex mixture of molecules with various combinations of the two possible heavy chains and two possible light chains. The products thus include significant amounts of bifunctional antibody containing one combining site characteristic of each parental cell (Milstein and Cuello, 1983). For normal purposes, good non-producing myeloma lines are now available for fusion, thus avoiding potential problems of product heterogeneity.

Several alternative strategies are possible after fusion in the effort to identify and isolate cell lines making the required antibody. We have preferred to plate cells initially into several hundred wells of microtitre trays. This approach presents a fairly formidable task for initial screening, but greatly facilitates the task of subsequent cloning. It also minimizes the risk of individual subcultures containing multiple positive hybrids, which can lead to confusion if antibodies are to be characterized before cloning. It is essential that screening assays are as rapid and simple as possible, and precise quantitation at this stage is unnecessary so long as specific antibody production can be identified. The type of screening assay used will depend on the nature, purity and quantity of antigen available, and many different variations are possible (Galfre and Milstein, 1981; Soos and Siddle, 1982; Elfman et al., 1985).

Once positive cultures have been identified, some preliminary characterization of antibody is desirable before too much effort is expended in cloning and growing cells which produce antibody of indifferent quality and little practical value. This screening is particularly important if fusions are very successful, requiring priorities to be established for processing a multitude of different cell lines. An estimate of antibody affinity and specificity at an early stage is always valuable, though once again these assessments need not be very precise. Some workers have recommended determination of antibody titres in culture fluids as a measure of relative affinity (van Heyningen et al., 1983), but this variable depends heavily on similarity in cell concentrations and antibody secretion rates, and the result could be very unreliable. Thus a very high titre may well be suggestive of a promising antibody, but a low titre at some stage does not necessarily indicate a poor product. Scatchard analysis in our view allows a more reliable, albeit still approximate, determination of antibody affinity (Soos and Siddle, 1982, 1983). We have sometimes in this way identified antibodies of high avidity, but low concentration, which might have been discounted on the basis of titre alone. Specificity of antibodies may conveniently be assessed by testing the relative titre for binding of labelled antigen and of appropriate labelled cross-reactants (Hunter et al., 1983; Soos and Siddle, 1983). A better quantitative estimate of relative binding affinities is obtained by comparing the potencies of unlabelled antigen, and cross-reactants in competing with labelled antigen in a conventional radioimmunoassay format (Soos and Siddle, 1982, 1983).

The desirability of spending time on the characterization of antibody at an early stage must be weighed against the need to proceed quickly with cloning potentially useful cell lines, to avoid possible overgrowth by non-producing cells. It is always possible, if necessary, to freeze some cells and to return to assess them later. Once a first cloning has been accomplished, the pace of work can usually be relaxed. We routinely reclone cells at least once more, to confirm monoclonality and stability of cell lines before growth in bulk for frozen storage and antibody production.

2.3. Antibody production and purification

The capacity for the production of polyclonal antibodies is always limited by the amount of serum which can be obtained at any one bleed, the extent of continued response to repeated immunization, and ultimately by the lifetime of the animal. Monoclonal antibody production knows no such limitations, and is restricted only by the scale of operation which the experimenter is prepared to undertake. Moreover, because hybrid myeloma cells may be stored in liquid nitrogen, repeated batches of unchanging antibody may be produced as required.

Two routes are available for the large-scale production of antibodies. One involves growing cells *in vitro*, and harvesting the antibodies from culture fluids. Much effort is being given to developing processes for large-scale cell culture in defined media, and some companies now advertise the production of tens of grams of antibody in this way. On the laboratory scale, targets must be more modest, but it should still be possible to obtain litre quantities of spent culture medium containing antibody in the concentration range 10–100 μg ml^{-1}. The alternative method of antibody production is to grow cells as intraperitoneal (ascites) tumours in animals, and to collect the tumour fluid and serum. Tumours will only grow in animals of the same species and inbred strain as that from which the lymphocytes and myeloma were derived. Antibody is present in tumour fluid at concentrations of 1–10 mg ml^{-1}, and 10 ml or more of such fluid may be obtained from a mouse by serial tapping. The preparation of gram quantities of monoclonal antibody *in vivo* therefore presents no great difficulties, though the large-scale induction of tumours for this purpose is undesirable.

The method of antibody production which is chosen will depend on the proposed use, the facilities available, the quantities of antibody and the degree of purity which are ultimately required. For example, antibodies intended for *in vivo* administration to man must meet the most rigorous standards of purity, which may be difficult to achieve with antibody obtained from animals.

For many of the familiar applications of antibodies in diagnostic immunoassay, no purification procedures are required. Thus in both competitive radioimmunoassay and methods dependent on precipitation, polyclonal antibodies have often been used simply in the form of diluted crude serum, or at best as a salt-fractionated total immunoglobulin preparation. This application is possible because such methods depend only on the functional and not the chemical purity of antibody.

In contrast, immunometric (labelled antibody) assay methods rely heavily on the availability of purified antibody, most especially for labelling, but also for the preparation of high capacity solid-phase reagents. This requirement has been a major factor limiting the development of immunometric assays when using polyclonal antisera. Specific antibodies in such sera can only be separated from total immunoglobulin by affinity techniques using immobilized antigen (Hales and Woodhead, 1980). This approach may also be used in the subfractionation of heterogeneous polyclonal sera to obtain antibody populations with different affinities or specificities (Hodgkinson and Lowry, 1982). It must be emphasized that in no way do such relatively crude subfractions of polyclonal sera approach monoclonality, as it is likely that hundreds or even thousands of antibodies differing in affinity and epitope are produced *in vivo*, directed against even quite simple antigens.

The purification of specific antibody from polyclonal sera suffers from two major difficulties. First, to obtain antibody in reasonable amounts, considerable quantities of purified antigen are necessary (approximately equal to the mass of antibody required) for production of the affinity reagent. The potential for re-use of affinity reagent only partially overcomes this problem. Second, the conditions used for the elution of specific antibody from the affinity reagent, such as extremes of pH, may damage its immunological activity, or, if less vigorous, fail to recover the antibody population of highest avidity. In addition, each antibody–antigen combination has to be studied individually to discover optimal elution conditions.

Monoclonal antibodies, in contrast, may easily be obtained at a purity more than adequate for use in diagnostic assays. The highest purity is potentially most easily obtained with antibody produced in culture fluids *in vitro*, as this process avoids the problem of removal of some non-immune immunoglobulin which is always present in tumour fluids generated *in vivo*. Ion-exchange chromatography, facilitated if necessary by prior salt fractionation, is an effective purification procedure which readily yields antibody of greater than 80% purity (Bruck *et al.*, 1982; Parham *et al.*, 1982), including removal of much of the contaminating non-immune immunoglobulin where present. Methods which effectively produce a total immunoglobulin fraction, including salt precipitation, or affinity chromatography with protein A, are particularly valuable for purifying antibody from culture fluids, where it is the only immunoglobulin present. These methods may also be adequate for many purposes even with tumour fluids, depending on the ratio of specific antibody to total immunoglobulin. However, not all mouse and rat antibodies react well with protein A.

The greater purity which may be achieved with monoclonal compared to polyclonal antibodies is an important factor contributing to their better performance as labelled reagents in immunometric assays. Thus monoclonal antibodies often give lower non-specific binding and higher specific binding than their polyclonal counterparts, improving both assay sensitivity and working range (Gray *et al.*, 1984).

3. PROPERTIES OF MONOCLONAL ANTIBODIES

Monoclonal antibodies are not inherently different from the antibodies which make up polyclonal antisera. Serum antibodies are only mixtures of monoclonal antibodies, albeit very complex and heterogeneous ones containing perhaps thousands of different molecules reacting with a given antigen, together with a large excess of non-immune immunoglobulin. One consequence of this complexity of serum antibodies is their variability between animals, and even during a course of immunization in a given animal. In contrast, the properties of a monoclonal antibody are by definition fixed and unchanging.

Some of the properties of antisera reflect the effects of averaging the behaviour of many different antibodies, or of synergistic or co-operative behaviour dependent on the simultaneous presence of multiple antibodies. As a result, polyclonal and monoclonal antibodies do show some significant differences in properties. Thus a minority of monoclonal antibodies might show unusual physical properties, such as sensitivity to pH, oxidizing agents or salt concentration, or be particularly susceptible to damage when iodinated or adsorbed on surfaces, whereas such effects on a subpopulation of serum antibodies would pass unnoticed against a mainly stable background. The vast majority of monoclonal antibodies are, however, very stable molecules, as are immunoglobulins in general.

Some properties of antibodies depend on isotype, or the particular class or subclass of heavy chain which they contain. Because monoclonal antibodies by definition possess only a single type of heavy chain, they do not all react well with complement or with protein A. In addition, the conditions for fragmentation of immunoglobulins to give Fab or $F(ab')_2$ structures depend on isotype, and thus vary for different monoclonal antibodies (Parham *et al.*, 1982). Class- and subclass-specific antisera are available which allow the easy identification of the isotype of mouse monoclonal antibodies. The frequency with which different isotypes are encountered will reflect their relative incidence *in vivo*. The mouse produces predominantly IgG_1 antibodies in secondary immune responses, but a relatively high frequency of IgM antibodies may be obtained in fusions following only a primary immunization. Other classes of antibody occur with lower frequency.

A further general difference between monoclonal and polyclonal antibodies is that monoclonals will not individually precipitate antigens unless these possess repeat epitopes. This characteristic is because bivalency of antibody and at least trivalency of antigen are required to form a three-dimensional precipitation lattice. When human IgG is the antigen, possessing by symmetry two copies of each epitope, mixtures of as few as two monoclonal antibodies are effective for precipitation (Deverill et al., 1981). It should in general be possible to produce defined precipitating mixtures from three or more monoclonal antibodies when antigens possess only a single copy of each epitope.

A further consequence of the fact that monoclonal antibodies recognize only a single epitope on an antigen is that they are less likely than polyclonal antibodies to inhibit function, such as the catalytic activity of enzymes or receptor binding of hormones. Monoclonal antibodies may therefore be useful reagents for the immunoextraction of isoenzymes from complex mixtures prior to assay (Bailyes et al., 1985), and in studying the orientation of hormones when bound to their receptors (Moyle et al., 1982).

3.1. Affinity

The affinity of monoclonal antibodies (or more correctly their avidity, if studied under conditions other than a simple bimolecular reaction) is frequently reported as being low relative to their polyclonal counterparts. As a result, some monoclonal antibodies cannot be used to produce assays with the necessary sensitivity for diagnostic use at low concentrations of analytes such as polypeptide hormones and tumour markers. This preponderance of low affinity monoclonal antibodies in part reflects the distribution of affinities seen in vivo, and even in polyclonal antisera of apparent high avidity the effective antibodies may represent only a small proportion of the total binding activity. We have determined affinity constants of monoclonal antibodies for various polypeptide antigens by Scatchard analysis, and found values as high as $10^{11} \, l \, mol^{-1}$, with a broad distribution down to $10^8 \, l \, mol^{-1}$ or less (Soos and Siddle, 1982, 1983; Morgan et al., 1984; Soos et al., 1984; Gard et al., 1985; Gray et al., 1985). These findings emphasize the need to look at large numbers of different antibodies in the pursuit of reagents for highly sensitive assays. It should not be forgotten, however, that even low affinity antibodies do have their uses, and are generally more suitable than their high affinity counterparts for use in immunopurification schemes (Morgan et al., 1983) because of the relative ease of elution of antigen in an active form.

Some recent evidence has suggested that the high avidity of polyclonal relative to monoclonal antibodies may reflect more than a simple statistical incidence of different individual affinities in a large population. Some mixtures of two monoclonal antibodies for different epitopes on a given

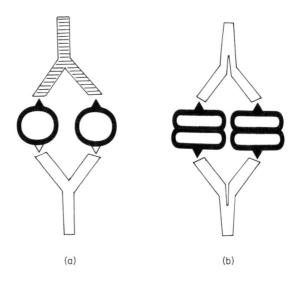

(a)   (b)

Fig. 1. Proposed structures of high avidity antibody–antigen complexes: (a) complex containing antigen with one copy of each epitope, and two different monoclonal antibodies; (b) complex containing dimeric antigen with two copies of each epitope, and two molecules of a single monoclonal antibody in which inter-chain disulphide bonds have been cleaved by reduction

antigen show co-operativity in that the avidity of the mixture is considerably higher than that of the individual antibodies. This phenomenon depends on antibody bivalency, and has been attributed to the formation of multimeric heterocyclic complexes (Fig. 1) containing two antigen molecules with appropriately oriented epitopes, and two different antibody molecules. It is envisaged that the high avidity of antigen binding in such complexes reflects the fact that antigen is attached simultaneously to more than one antibody, rather than any change in the affinity of interaction at any one epitope (Ehrlich *et al.*, 1983; Holmes and Parham, 1983; Thompson and Jackson, 1984). However, alternative mechanisms for enhancement of the binding of one antibody by a second antibody appear to occur in other instances, involving conformational changes induced or stabilized by one antibody so as to favour binding of the other to a modified epitope (Thompson and Jackson, 1984).

We have encountered an example of enhanced avidity of a single mono-clonal antibody dependent on the formation of multimolecular aggregates. A group of antibodies directed against one particular epitope on the homo-dimeric protein, brain-type creatine kinase (CK-BB), were found to show up to a 50-fold increase in avidity for CK-BB after the reduction of inter-heavy chain disulphide bonds. This treatment did not affect the overall integrity of the native antibody, but apparently increased molecular flexibility sufficiently to allow formation of cyclic complexes of high avidity containing two dimeric antigen molecules and two identical antibody molecules (Jackson *et al.*, 1983). The phenomenon was relatively specific and was not shown by antibodies to other epitopes on CK-BB, nor by any antibodies in their reaction with the heart-type heterodimer CK-MB. This finding presumably reflects the steric constraints imposed by the orientation of the various epitopes, and by the requirement for antigen bivalency in forming complexes with a single monoclonal antibody (Fig. 1).

It appears from these results that the best way to produce high avidity reagents from monoclonal antibodies may be by judicious mixing to generate defined and reproducible 'oligoclonal' antibodies. The accompanying use of disulphide bond reductants may allow further enhancement, or extend the range of mixtures which show such effects. It also seems likely that the high avidity of conventional polyclonal antisera results in part from autoselection of appropriate antibody combinations to generate high avidity complexes. This explanation could also account for the relatively long times required (sometimes days at 4°C) for polyclonal sera to reach binding equilibrium with antigen at low concentrations. Monoclonal antibodies in our experience achieve equilibrium very much more rapidly (at most a few hours), presumably reflecting a simpler bimolecular reaction under most conditions.

3.2. Specificity

The fine specificity of antibodies is a very important consideration when they are required to assay individual polypeptides or haptens in the presence of potentially cross-reacting compounds with common epitopes, whether these are degradation products or naturally occurring homologues. In principle monoclonal antibodies may be obtained for unique epitopes on a given antigen. This situation is much harder to achieve for polyclonal antibodies which usually bind to multiple sites on an antigen, and occur as a complex mixture which is difficult to resolve except by repeated adsorption or affinity purification with potential cross-reactants or fragments of antigen.

The powers of discrimination of monoclonal antibodies are considerable, and are well illustrated in the case of some antibodies we have obtained for human chorionic gonadotrophin (hCG)(Table 2). This hormone shares a common α subunit with human thyrotropin (TSH) and human lutropin (LH), and also shows approx. 80% β subunit homology with LH. Nevertheless, monoclonal antibodies with high specificity for hCG are readily obtained (Gard *et al.*, 1985), as well as antibodies which cross-react strongly with LH. Moreover, some antibodies react only with the intact $\alpha\beta$ structure and not with free subunits, while others react preferably with free β-subunit although obtained by immunization with intact molecule. When β-subunit was used as

Table 2. Cross-reactivity of antibodies for hCG

Antibody code	Affinity (1 mol^{-1})		Relative affinity (%)				
	hCG	β-hCG	hCG	β-hCG	LH	TSH	FSH
1/3	—	2×10^{10}	30	100	10	< 1	7
2/6	—	1×10^{10}	< 1	100	< 1	< 1	< 1
3/6	6×10^9	—	100	1600	2	< 1	< 1
9/7	4×10^9	—	100	< 1	5	1	< 1
11/6	2×10^{11}	—	100	< 1	40	3	4
12/17	6×10^{10}	—	100	120	1	< 1	< 1

Relative affinities were calculated from potency in competitive immunoassays using ^{125}I-labelled hCG or ^{125}I-labelled β-hCG free subunit as tracer, and are expressed relative to affinity for immunogen with each antibody. Actual affinities were calculated from binding equilibrium at 0°C by Scatchard analysis. Data from Gard et al. (1985).

immunogen, many of the monoclonal antibodies obtained reacted only with free subunit and not at all with intact molecule. These results indicate a substantial dependence of epitope accessibility or conformation on the state of assembly of this particular hormone.

We have had similar results with monoclonal antibodies for a variety of different antigens. Thus, several antibodies raised against the brain-type isoenzyme of creatine kinase (CK-BB) reacted only with the homodimer BB, and not with the heterodimer MB (Jackson et al., 1984). It is not yet clear whether the epitope concerned is a 'bridge' region between two subunits, or reflects a conformational difference between B subunits in the two isoenzymes. We have not so far detected analogous antibodies showing specificity only for the MB isoenzyme, but have several antibodies for BB or MM (muscle) isoenzymes which also bind to the corresponding subunit in the MB heterodimer.

Recently we have made several monoclonal antibodies for human proinsulin (Gray et al., 1985). This hormone is synthesized as a single polypeptide chain and cleaved internally at two sites to remove C-peptide and leave the disulphide-linked A and B chains of insulin. We have one antibody which is relatively specific for intact proinsulin and another which binds preferentially to one of the partially proteolysed forms as well as to the intact molecule. Yet another antibody reacts almost equally with all forms of proinsulin and with insulin. These antibodies should enable us to investigate the pathway of processing of proinsulin in vivo, and the nature of circulating proinsulin in human sera. Previous polyclonal antisera raised against proinsulin or C-peptide have lacked the necessary fine specificity for such studies to be attempted.

Other workers have described monoclonal antibodies specific for different size variants of growth hormone (Wallis *et al.*, 1982), allelic variants of placental alkaline phosphatase (Slaughter *et al.*, 1981) and individual steroid hormones (Kohen *et al.*, 1982). It is clear, therefore, that the powers of discrimination of monoclonal antibodies are potentially very great, though impossible to predict in advance. The ability to obtain highly specific antibodies obviously depends on the existence of structural features unique to a given molecule, and on the maximum affinity differences likely to be possible to allow binding to these, but not to modified epitopes on other molecules. It is also necessary that such structural features make a significant contribution to the overall immunogenicity of the molecule. This requirement may not always be the case. Thus, the isoenzymes of alkaline phosphatase from human liver and bone have some differences in physical properties which presumably have their basis in a structural difference, of amino acid sequence or post-translational modification. All the monoclonal antibodies which we (Bailyes *et al.*, 1985) and others (Meyer *et al.*, 1982) have so far prepared for the liver isoenzyme have failed to discriminate this antigen from the bone isoenzyme. Presumably the dominant epitopes are common to both isoenzymes in this case. Similarly, attempts to prepare monoclonal antibodies capable of discriminating between carcinoembryonic antigen (CEA) and normal cross-reacting antigens (NCA) have so far been disappointing (Hedin *et al.*, 1983).

The dependence of recognition by monoclonal antibody on a single epitope might be seen as a disadvantage if the possibility exists of polymorphism at that epitope which is not important for biological activity or diagnostic measurement. Assays based on a monoclonal antibody in such a situation might underestimate antigen concentration under some conditions, whereas reactivity of the same antigen with a polyclonal antibody capable of binding at multiple epitopes could provide a better measure of overall immunoreactivity. Polymorphism of antigen could result from physical or chemical changes during sample handling or storage (hence the concept of an especially 'labile' epitope), or might occur endogenously as a consequence of differences in post-translational modification or processing in different physiological or pathological states. This phenomenon has not in practice proved a problem in the use of monoclonal antibodies. Presumably such occurrences are relatively rare, or have little effect on the majority of epitopes in a given antigen. If antibodies are identified which discriminate between minor structural variants, these may be used to advantage to investigate the physiological basis and significance of such changes.

3.3. Epitope Analysis

It is frequently important in the application of monoclonal antibodies to identify pairs of antibodies which are able to bind simultaneously to spatially distinct epitopes on a given antigen, without mutual steric hindrance. This is necessary, for instance, in the development of two-site immunometric assays, and in the preparation of co-operative or precipitating antibody mixtures. Differences in the fine specificity of antibodies, though indicative of different epitopes, do not guarantee that such epitopes are well separated in space so as to accommodate binding of the respective very large antibody molecules. It is necessary, therefore, to test for competition in binding of different antibodies to a given antigen. In general, the larger the antigen, the greater will be the number of 'independent' epitopes. We have identified three separate antigenic regions associated with the β-subunit of TSH of M_r–15 000 daltons (Soos et al., 1984), and with proinsulin of M_r–19 000 daltons (Gray et al., 1985). We have no experience of smaller peptides, but have heard verbal reports of two-site binding to peptides of M_r–2000 daltons. This size corresponds to only 18 amino acids, and when it is considered that the antibody combining site accommodates structures of the size of a pentapeptide, this must be about the lower theoretical limit for simultaneous two-site binding. It is generally assumed that haptens such as steroids are too small to permit binding of two antibodies simultaneously, but it is not inconceivable that antibodies generated to suitable different conjugates might make this possible.

As suggested earlier, some epitopes in polypeptides may be 'conformational', consisting of amino acid residues from different parts of a polypeptide chain which are brought into proximity in the native tertiary structure. In other cases, epitopes present in intact molecules may also be identified in short peptides derived from these molecules. This observation provides a method of analysis of antigenic regions where a complete amino acid sequence is known and various fragments are available. We have recently studied monoclonal antibodies for human myelin basic protein (MBP) from this point of view (Elfman et al., 1985). This information may in turn be used to analyse the relative orientation of epitopes in the native protein structure, for example in the identification of peptide sequences which are exposed at the external cell surface in membrane proteins such as MBP.

4. APPLICATIONS OF MONOCLONAL ANTIBODIES

Polyclonal antisera have found widespread diagnostic applications in assays based on precipitation of antigen (immunodiffusion, immunoelectrophoresis, nephelometry) and on competitive binding of labelled and unlabelled antigen (radio-, fluoro- and enzyme-immunoassay). Precipitation methods depend on the ability of mixtures of bivalent antibodies to cross-link antigen molecules into three-dimensional lattices. This is not a property shared by individual monoclonal antibodies, but may be obtained with mixtures. Competitive methods, which are potentially much more sensitive, depend on the high avidity of polyclonal antibodies, favouring binding of antigen even when both reactants are present at low concentrations. In fact it is the avidity of the antibody which ultimately limits the sensitivity achievable in competitive assays (Ekins, Chapter 13 in this volume). Only a small proportion of monoclonal antibodies have avidities comparable to the best polyclonals, although once again the use of mixed monoclonals may be beneficial in this context. Monoclonal antibodies may also be of value in non-isotopic immunoassays for haptens to ensure that the labelled antigen and analyte compete for the same binding sites.

A third type of method, to which monoclonal antibodies have much to contribute, is the immunometric assay. In this technique, labelled antibody added in excess is reacted with antigen and the amount of bound label provides a direct measure of antigen concentration (Woodhead et al., 1974). A separation step is necessary in order to determine the amount of labelled antibody bound, and this objective is most easily achieved by using a second specific antibody, coupled to solid phase, which can bind to antigenic sites not occupied by labelled antibody (Fig. 2). As with competitive assay methods a variety of different labels have been employed (most usually ^{125}I in the immunoradiometric assay, IRMA). Many variations in detailed assay protocol are possible, notably in the timing and order of addition of the labelled and solid phase antibody reagents.

It has come to be recognized that two-site immunometric assays have considerable advantages over competitive immunoassay methods, both in theory and practice (Hunter and Budd, 1981; Ekins, Chapter 13 in this volume). Thus, immunometric assays offer a wider effective working range with good precision, and a linear response for a considerable dose range, which allows single-point calibration for some applications. Most importantly, immunometric methods are capable of greater sensitivity, given a labelled antibody of sufficiently high specific activity and low non-specific binding. In theory this sensitivity is not limited by the avidity of the labelled antibody, as

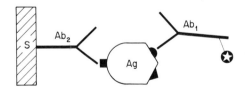

Fig. 2. Principle of the two-site immunometric assay. The components of the assay are a labelled antibody (Ab_1) directed against one epitope, and a second antibody (Ab_2) directly or indirectly linked to the solid phase (S) and directed against a second distinct epitope. Specific association of label with solid phase occurs only in the presence of antigen (Ag) and provides a direct measure of antigen concentration

the reaction is favoured by excess reagent conditions. An antibody of given avidity will thus produce a more sensitive assay in an immunometric than in a competitive format, although it is always an advantage to use the antibody of highest available avidity in both these techniques. The reaction times necessary to produce sensitive immunometric assays are generally much shorter than for competitive methods, again reflecting the use of excess rather than limiting antibody concentration. Two-site assays may also possess enhanced specificity for intact molecules, because of the dependence of assay response on the simultaneous recognition of at least two epitopes by different antibody molecules. A final practical advantage of immunometric methods lies in the ease of labelling of antibodies, by techniques which are in principle the same for all assays, as contrasted with the labelling of antigens where each may bring its own problems. The only major limitation inherent in the two-site immunometric assay is the requirement for an antigen of sufficient size and with appropriately oriented epitopes to permit binding of at least two antibodies. This method cannot therefore be used in the assay of haptens and small peptides.

To date the application of immunometric assays in diagnostic laboratories has been very limited. This situation reflects the serious practical difficulties in realizing the theoretical advantages of the technique when working with polyclonal antibodies. Thus, it is necessary to use purified antibody for labelling, and preferably also for coupling to solid phase. Two different antibodies must normally be used which do not significantly compete for binding sites on the antigen. The amounts of antibody required are also much greater than for competitive assays. The advent of monoclonal antibodies solves all these problems, as will be readily appreciated from the foregoing account of their purification and properties. Moreover, even antibodies of only moderate affinity will produce useful immunometric assays when a competitive immunoassay with the same antibody would be too insensitive to be of value (Weeks et al., 1981). Immunometric assays employing monoclonal antibodies for several polypeptide antigens have been described recently, making use of a variety of different labels, solid phases and assay protocols (reviewed in Siddle, 1984, 1985). Examples from our own work will be used to illustrate some of the factors to be considered in the design of immunometric assays, many of which are not dependent on the nature of individual analytes.

4.1. Immunometric assay of TSH

We have produced and characterized a large number of monoclonal antibodies for TSH, including some which possess both excellent specificity and very high affinity, and which bind to three distinct epitopes (Soos et al., 1984). Initially these antibodies were evaluated using antibody-coated plastic tubes as solid phase and ^{125}I as label. This assay format was convenient for the comparison of different antibody combinations and concentrations, because of the ease of preparation of both solid phase and labelled antibody. This approach allowed the selection of optimal antibody combinations for use in more sophisticated assay formats. Although antibody excess may theoretically be used to maximize binding to antigen, the non-specific binding of labelled antibody to solid phase may become unacceptably high if too much labelled antibody is added. This results in loss of precision at low antigen concentrations and poorer assay sensitivity. For this reason it is important to use the antibody of highest available affinity for labelling, so that the binding to antigen approaches a maximum without the need for too high an antibody concentration. In the case of TSH, we were fortunate to have antibodies with affinity constants approaching 10^{11} l mol^{-1}, which allowed very sensitive assays to be established. A detection limit for TSH of 10^{-16} mol in the assay was readily achieved, albeit corresponding to a count rate of less than 100 cts min^{-1} (Soos et al., 1984).

For routine diagnostic use, a modified assay protocol was adopted, in which antibody was covalently coupled to aminocellulose (Hales and Woodhead, 1980) for use as a solid-phase reagent. This material had a high binding capacity, was easily pipetted and conveniently separated by filtration on a Kemtek 3000 automated immunoassay machine for the determination of bound radioactivity. An additional advantage was that a two-step assay protocol was possible in which the sample was preincubated with ^{125}I-labelled antibody before addition of solid phase. This speeds the overall reaction, allowing a sensitive assay (detection limit 0.2–0.3 mIU l^{-1}) with a total incubation time of only 4 h. Results on patient samples showed excellent agreement with a conventional RIA used previously, which took 3 days to perform and was less sensitive (S. Olpin, P. Raggatt, J. Burrin and K. Siddle, unpublished results).

A further development of the immunometric technique is shown in Fig. 3. In this system a mixture of two different ^{125}I-labelled monoclonal antibodies is used to maximize the amount of label which can be specifically bound to TSH. These antibodies are directed against different epitopes both specific for intact TSH. A third antibody for yet another epitope is not directly linked to solid phase, but instead conjugated to fluorescein. This reagent allows rapid reaction in solution phase of all three antibodies, followed by a brief reaction with a solid-phase polyclonal anti-fluorescein isothiocyanate (FITC) antibody (Rattle et al., 1984). The last reaction is rapid and of high avidity because of the multiple fluorescein molecules attached to each antibody molecule. The use of magnetizable cellulose (Forrest and Rattle, 1983) as the solid-phase matrix provides a clean and rapid basis for separation and washing, and a very low non-specific binding of labelled antibody. As a result, the detection limit in this assay is less than 0.15 mIU l^{-1}, with a linear response over the whole clinically significant range up to 30 mIU l^{-1}, and a total assay time of only 2 h (Fig. 4).

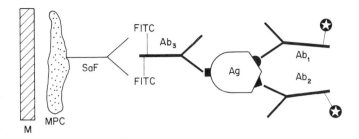

Fig. 3. Immunometric assay modified to increase sensitivity and enhance reaction kinetics. The assay contains two different ^{125}I-labelled antibodies for distinct epitopes (Ab_1, Ab_2) and an FITC-conjugated antibody for a third epitope (Ab_3). The cocktail of these antibodies is incubated in solution with antigen before addition of solid-phase reagent which consists of sheep anti-FITC antibody (SαF) coupled to magnetic particle-cellulose (MPC). Separation and washing are achieved with the aid of a magnet (M) placed under the reaction tubes at the end of the incubation. [Courtesy of Drs Simon Rattle and Gordon Forrest, Serono Diagnostics Ltd, Woking, U.K.]

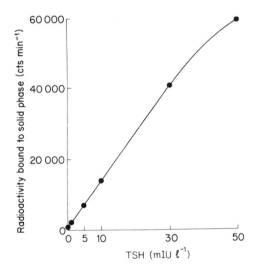

Fig. 4. Dose-response curve for immunoradiometric assay of TSH. The assay format is as shown in Fig. 3. A cocktail of ^{125}I-labelled antibodies D88 and E21 (approx. 2×10^5 cts min^{-1} and FITC-conjugated D49 (100 μl) was incubated with serum sample or standard at the concentrations shown (200 μl) for 2 h. A suspension of anti-FITC magnetizable particles (200 μl) was added for a further 5 min before sedimentation and washing using a magnetic separator, and measurement of radioactivity in the resultant pellet. The within-assay coefficient of variation is better than 10% at 0.5 mIU l^{-1}, and the detection limit of the assay is approx. 0.15 mIU l^{-1}. One milli-IU is approximately equivalent to 0.17 μg or 6 pmol of TSH. [Courtesy of Drs Simon Rattle and Gordon Forrest, Serono Diagnostics Ltd, Woking, UK]

Given monoclonal antibodies of high avidity, and a solid phase with a sufficiently low non-specific binding of labelled antibody, the detection limit of the immunometric assay is ultimately limited by the specific radioactivity of ^{125}I-labelled antibody. Further improvements in sensitivity are possible only by the use of labels which provide a greater measurable signal per unit mass of antibody. One such label is a chemiluminescent acridinium ester (Weeks *et al.*, 1983). This reagent can be used to give specific activities in terms of 10^6 photon counts per nanogram of labelled antibody (Weeks *et al.*, 1984), compared to some 10^4 radioactive counts per minute per nanogram achieved with ^{125}I. The chemiluminescent-labelled antibody can be used in an im-munochemiluminometric assay (ICMA) for TSH with an antigen detection limit below 0.01 mIU l^{-1}, or approximately 5×10^{-18} mol in the assay. This ultrasensitive assay has for the first time allowed a clear distinction between TSH levels in thyrotoxic and euthyroid subjects (Weeks *et al.*, 1984).

An alternative approach which yields an assay of similarly high sensitivity is the amplified ELISA (Fig. 5). The principle of amplification by enzymatic cycling reactions is well known in biochemistry, but has not been previously applied to immunoassay. The technique provides a 100-fold increase in measurable absorbance for a given amount of enzyme-labelled antibody

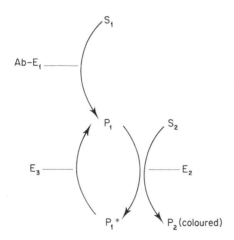

Fig. 5. Principle of the amplified ELISA. Antibody is conjugated to an enzyme E_1 which catalyses the conversion of substrate S_1 to product P_1 in a first reaction incubation. Amplifier solution is then added containing enzyme E_2 which converts S_2 to P_2, using P_1 as a cofactor. Enzyme E_3 regenerates P_1 and so allows each molecule of P_1 generated in the first reaction to participate in the formation of many molecules of P_2. As a result, the eventual colour generated by P_2 can be amplified approximately 100-fold in a given reaction time compared to the direct assay of E_1 with a chromogenic substrate. [Courtesy of Dr Axel Johannsson, IQ (Bio) Ltd., Cambridge, U.K.]

within a given reaction time. The double amplification effect of the two sequential enzyme reactions allows the relatively insensitive technique of spectrophotometry, quantitating coloured product in the 10^{-6} mol l^{-1} concentration range, to provide an accurate measure of TSH at concentrations below 10^{-13} mol l^{-1} (Fig. 6). Although the assay sensitivity is therefore comparable to that achieved by luminescent labelling, the working range is narrower because of the upper limit imposed by spectrophotometric detection. This limitation is compensated for by the convenience of the detection system. The use of antibody-coated microtitre trays as solid phase permits rapid, simultaneous quantitation of 96 sample wells using multichannel micro-ELISA photometers.

Each of the TSH assay techniques discussed has its own advantages and limitations, but all produce highly sensitive and rapid assay methods. The use of ^{125}I for labelling is likely to remain dominant in the UK for some time, but the advantages of reagent stability and safety, and the potential for greater

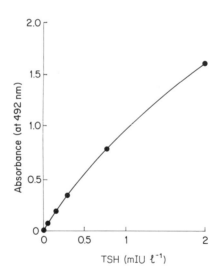

Fig. 6. Dose-response curve for assay of TSH by amplified ELISA. Antibody D88 conjugated to enzyme E_1 (75 µl) was incubated with serum sample or standard at the concentrations shown (25 µl) in the wells of plastic microtitre trays which had been previously coated with antibody D49. After 2 h, the wells were washed, and substrate S_1 added. After reaction for 20 min, amplifier solution ($E_2 + E_3 + S_2$) was added for a further 10 min, before stopping the reaction and reading absorbance at 492 nm on a Multiscan photometer. The within-assay coefficient of variation is better than 10% at 0.05 mIU/l^{-1}, and the detection limit of the assay is approximately 0.01 mIU/l^{-1}. [Courtesy of Dr. Axel Johannsson, IQ (Bio) Ltd, Cambridge, U.K.]

sensitivity, indicate that non-isotopic labels such as enzymes and luminescent compounds will find increasingly important applications in the future.

4.2. Other two-site assays

Other aspects and variants of two-site assay methods are illustrated by some recent work on assays for hCG and creatine kinase. Antibodies to hCG (Table 2) have been used to establish assays specific for intact molecule, free β-subunit, or total β-subunit respectively (Gard et al., 1985; Rattle et al., 1984). Previous radioimmunoassays have probably detected both intact molecule and free subunit, though not necessarily with equal potency. The availability of high avidity monoclonal antibodies once again allows the development of a two-site immunoradiometric assay which provides sensitivity of better than 0.1 ng ml^{-1} in an assay time which can be as short as 15 min (Rattle et al., 1984). One problem in the assay of hCG is the extremely wide range of concentrations (at least four orders of magnitude) which may be encountered physiologically. This necessitates either the use of two-step assay procedures or of high antibody concentrations, to avoid potential problems arising from antigen excess (Nomura et al., 1982).

Similar difficulties of slightly different origin were encountered in the assay of the MB isoenzyme of creatine kinase from heart (Jackson et al., 1984). This assay made use of a solid-phase antibody to the M subunit and an iodinated antibody to the B subunit, and was therefore potentially susceptible to interference from MM and BB isoenzymes present in samples—often in excess over MB. Although neither of the homodimers can give a positive assay response, they will compete with MB for available antibody and so possibly lead to underestimation of MB concentration. Once again, two-step protocols and excess antibody concentrations can overcome this problem, in the latter case with some sacrifice in terms of assay sensitivity.

A totally different form of interference in two-site assays can arise from the presence of anti-immunoglobulin antibodies in human serum. These may be produced initially as a response to bovine immunoglobulin in milk, but cross-react with antibodies from a variety of species. The incidence of such antibodies may be as high as 7% when working with polyclonal sheep antisera, but is certainly much less in mouse monoclonal systems (Hunter et al., 1983). We have encountered occasional false high values in several different two-site assays which seem to be due to anti-mouse immunoglobulin activity cross-linking solid phase and labelled reagents independently of the presence of antigen (R. J. Thompson, P. Gray. G. M. Addison and K. Siddle, unpublished). Both non-immune mouse and sheep immunoglobulins added to the assays are usually effective in preventing this artefact. The incidence of such problems with two-site mouse monoclonal antibody assays applies to probably less than 1% of human serum samples.

4.3. Homogeneous (non-separation) immunometric assays

One of the goals of many immunoassay methods is the development of techniques to avoid a separation step in the quantitation of bound labelled antigen or antibody. This achievement would allow the development of simpler and shorter assays, which are more easily automated. As yet there has been rather little progress in this direction with two-site assays, but several approaches are possible.

We have used red cell-labelled monoclonal antibodies in the assay of hCG by reverse passive haemagglutination (Siddle *et al.*, 1984). Two different antibodies were separately attached to sheep erythrocytes, which were then stabilized with glutaraldehyde to allow long-term storage. Quantitation of antigen was achieved by end-point determination when serial dilutions of sample or standard were incubated with mixed red cells, the haemagglutination reaction being observed after settling under gravity for 90 min. This method has a sensitivity comparable to that of immunoradiometric assays using the same antibodies, and though by no means as precise, has the advantages of simplicity and independence from instrumentation (see Chapter 4 in this volume). The reverse passive haemagglutination assay may be particularly valuable for giving a rapid yes/no answer on samples tested at fixed dilution, as in pregnancy testing, or screening of tumour markers.

An alternative and more sophisticated approach to separation-free methodology is the proximal linkage assay. In this method it is envisaged that two monoclonal antibodies for different epitopes are suitably labelled to cause emission or quenching of a signal when simultaneous binding to antigen brings them into close proximity (Sevier *et al.*, 1981; Thompson, 1983). Such methods might be based, for instance, on fluorescence or chemiluminescence energy transfer (Campbell, Chapter 10 in this volume) or enzyme channelling, but have yet to be evaluated in detail. Success will depend in part on the ability to bind two antibodies with sufficient proximity for efficient signal generation or transfer to occur, but without steric hindrance to the binding reactions themselves. This objective should provide yet another area in which the great potential and versatility of highly selected monoclonal antibodies will be fruitfully exploited in the future.

ACKNOWLEDGEMENTS

I am indebted to many colleagues and collaborators for stimulating discussions and for much of the experimental work reviewed in this chapter, especially Maria Soos, Trevor Gard, Tony Jackson, Rod Thompson, Elaine Bailyes, Peter Gray and Professors Nick Hales and Robin Coombs in Cambridge, and Ian Weeks, Stuart Woodhead, Paul Morgan and Tony Campbell at the Welsh National School of Medicine in Cardiff. I am also very grateful for the support and encouragement this work has received from Serono Diagnostics Ltd, of Woking, and IQ (Bio) Ltd, of Cambridge, and particularly to Gordon Forrest and Chris Keightley respectively for their liberal attitudes to commercial support of academic departments. Last, but by no means least, I thank the Wellcome Trust for the award of a Wellcome Senior Lectureship, and for the support of my work in this and other areas.

REFERENCES

Bailyes, E. M., Siddle, K., and Luzio, J. P. (1985). Monoclonal antibodies against human alkaline phosphatases. *Biochem. Soc. Trans.* (in press).

Bastin, J. M., Kirkley, J. and McMichael, A. J. (1982). Production of monoclonal antibodies: a practical guide. In *Monoclonal Antibodies in Clinical Medicine* (A. J. McMichael and J. W. Fabre, eds), Academic Press, London, pp 503–517.

Bruck, C., Portetelle, D., Glineur, C., and Bollen, A. (1982). One-step purification of mouse monoclonal antibodies from ascitic fluid by DEAE–Affigel Blue chromatography. *J. Immunol. Meth.* **53**, 313–319.

Dalchau, R., and Fabre, J. W. (1982). The purification of antigens and other studies with monoclonal antibody affinity columns: the complementary new dimension of monoclonal antibodies. In *Monoclonal Antibodies in Clinical Medicine* (A. J. McMichael and J. W. Fabre, eds), Academic Press, London, pp 519–556.

Deverill, I., Jefferis, R., Ling, N. R. and Reeves, W. G. (1981). Monoclonal antibodies to human IgG: reaction characteristics in the centrifugal analyser. *Clin. Chem.* **27**, 2044–2047.

Ehrlich, P. H., Moyle, W. R. and Moustafa, Z. A. (1983). Further characterization of cooperative interactions of monoclonal antibodies. *J. Immunol.* **131**, 1906–1912.

Elfman, L., Kynoch, P. A. M., Siddle, K. and Thompson, R. J. (1985). Rat and mouse monoclonal antibodies to human myelin basic protein (in preparation).

Forrest, G. C. and Rattle, S. J. (1983). Magnetic particle radioimmunoassay. In *Immunoassays for Clinical Chemistry*, 2nd edn. (W. M. Hunter and J. E. T. Corrie, eds), Churchill-Livingstone, Edinburgh, pp. 147–162.

Galfre, G. and Milstein, C. (1981). Preparation of monoclonal antibodies: strategies and procedures. *Meth. Enzymol.* **73**, 3–46.

Gard, T., Soos, M., Taylor, S. J. and Siddle, K. (1985). Specific and sensitive immunoradiometric assays for HCG and its β-subunit, using monoclonal antibodies (in preparation).

Gray, I. P., Siddle, K., Docherty, K., Frank, B. H. and Hales, C. N. (1984). Proinsulin in human serum: problems in measurement and interpretation. *Clin. Endocr.* **21**, 43–47.

Gray, I. P., Siddle, K., Frank, B. H. and Hales, C. N. (1985) Characterization and use of monoclonal antibodies directed against human proinsulin (in preparation).

Hales, C. N. and Woodhead, J. S. (1980). Labelled antibodies and their use in the immunoradiometric assay. *Meth. Enzymol.* **70**, 334–355.

Hedin, A., Carlsson, L., Berglund, A. and Hammarstrom, S. (1983). A monoclonal antibody–enzyme immunoassay for serum carcinoembryonic antigen with increased specificity for carcinomas. *Proc. natn. Acad. Sci. U.S.A.* **80**, 3470–3474.

Hodgkinson, S. C. and Lowry, P. J. (1982). Selective elution of immunoadsorbed anti-(human prolactin) immunoglobulins with enhanced immunochemical properties. *Biochem. J.* **205**, 535–541.

Holmes, N. J. and Parham, P. (1983). Enhancement of monoclonal antibodies against HLA–A2 is due to antibody bivalency. *J. biol. Chem.* **258**, 1580–1586.

Hunter, W. M. and Budd, P. S. (1981). Immunoradiometric versus radioimmunoassay: a comparison using alpha-fetoprotein as the model analyte. *J. Immunol. Meth.* **45**, 255–273.

Hunter, W. M., Bennie, J. G., Budd, P. S., Van Heyningen, V., James, K., Micklem, R. L. and Scott, A. (1983). Immunoradiometric assays using monoclonal antibodies. In *Immunoassays for Clinical Chemistry*, 2nd edn (W. M. Hunter and J. E. T. Corrie eds), Churchill-Livingstone, Edinburgh, pp. 531–544.

Jackson, A. P., Siddle, K. and Thompson, R. J. (1983). A monoclonal antibody to human brain-type creatine kinase: increased avidity with mercaptans. *Biochem. J.* **215**, 505–512.

Jackson, A. P., Siddle, K. and Thompson, R. J. (1984). Two-site monoclonal antibody assays for human heart- and brain-type creatine kinase. *Clin. Chem.* **30**, 1157–1162.

Kohen, F., Lichter, S., Eshhar, Z. and Lindner, H. R. (1982). Preparation of monoclonal antibodies able to discriminate between testosterone and 5α-dihydrotestosterone. *Steroids* **39**, 453–459.

Meyer, L. J., Lafferty, M. A., Raducha, M. G., Foster, C. J., Gogolin, K. J. and Harris, H. (1982). Production of a monoclonal antibody to human liver alkaline phosphatase. *Clin. Chim. Acta* **126**, 109–117.

Milstein, C. and Cuello, C. (1983). Hybrid–hybrid myelomas and their use in immunohistochemistry. *Nature, Lond.* **305**, 537–540.

Morgan, B. P., Daw, R. A., Siddle, K., Luzio, J. P. and Campbell, A. K. (1984). Immunoaffinity purification of human complement component C9 using monoclonal antibodies. *J. Immunol. Meth.* **64**, 269–281.

Moyle, W. R., Ehrlich, P. H. and Canfield, R. E. (1982). Use of monoclonal antibodies to subunits of human chorionic gonadotropin to examine the orientation of the hormone in its complex with receptor. *Proc. natn. Acad. Sci. U.S.A.* **79**, 2245–2249.

Nomura, M., Imai, M., Usuda, S., Nakamura, T., Miyakawa, Y. and Mayumi, M. (1982). A pitfall in two-site sandwich 'one-step' immunoassay with monoclonal antibodies for the determination of human alpha-fetoprotein. *J. Immunol. Meth.* **56**, 13–17.

Parham, P., Androlewicz, M. J., Brodsky, F. M., Holmes, N. J. and Ways, J. P. (1982). Monoclonal antibodies: purification and application to structural and functional studies of class I MHC antigens. *J. Immunol. Meth.* **53**, 133–173.

Rattle, S. J., Purnell, D. R., Williams, P. I. M., Siddle, K. and Forrest, G. C. (1984). New separation method for monoclonal immunoradiometric assays and its application to assays for thyrotropin and human chorionic gonadotropin. *Clin. Chem.* **30**, 1457–1461.

Secher, D. S. and Burke, D. C. (1980). A monoclonal antibody for large-scale purification of human leukocyte interferon. *Nature, Lond.* **285**, 446–450.

Sevier, E. D., David, G. S., Martinis, J., Desmond, W. J., Bartholomew, R. M. and Wang, R. (1981). Monoclonal antibodies in clinical immunology. *Clin. Chem.* **27**, 1797–1806.

Siddle, K. (1984). Clinical assays of products of normal and malignant cells. *Br. med. Bull.* **40**, 276–282.

Siddle, K. (1985). Monoclonal antibodies in clinical biochemistry. *Rec. Adv. Clin. Biochem.* **3**, in press.

Siddle, K., Gard, T., Thomas, D., Cranage, M. P. and Coombs, R. R. A. (1984). Red cell-labelled monoclonal antibodies for assay of human chorionic gonadotropin and luteinizing hormone by reverse passive haemagglutination. *J. Immunol. Meth.* **73**, 169–176.

Slaughter, C. A., Coseo, M. C., Cancro, M. P. and Harris, H. (1981). Detection of enzyme polymorphism by using monoclonal antibodies. *Proc. natn. Acad. Sci. U.S.A.* **78**, 1124–1128.

Soos, M. and Siddle, K. (1982). Characterization of monoclonal antibodies directed against human thyroid stimulating hormone. *J. Immunol. Meth.* **51**, 57–68.

Soos, M. and Siddle, K. (1983). Characterization of monoclonal antibodies for human luteinizing hormone, and mapping of antigenic determinants on the hormone. *Clin. Chim. Acta* **133**, 263–274.

Soos, M., Taylor, S. J., Gard, T. and Siddle, K. (1984). A rapid, sensitive two-site immunometric assay for TSH using monoclonal antibodies: investigation of factors affecting optimisation. *J. Immunol. Meth.* **73**, 237–249.

Stähli, C., Staehelin, T., Miggiano, V., Schmidt, J. and Häring, P. (1980). High frequencies of antigen-specific hybridomas: dependence on immunization parameters and prediction by spleen cell analysis. *J. Immunol. Meth.* **32**, 297–304.

Thompson, R. J. (1983). Are monoclonal antibodies the end of radioimmunoassay? *Trends biochem. Sci.* **7**, 419–420.

Thompson, R. J. and Jackson, A. P. (1984). Cyclic complexes and high avidity antibodies. *Trends biochem. Sci.* **9**, 1–3.

Van Heyningen, V., Brock, D. J. and Van Heyningen, S. (1983). A simple method for ranking the affinities of monoclonal antibodies. *J. Immunol. Meth.* **62**, 147–153.

Wallis, M., Ivanyi, T. K. and Surowy, T. K. (1982). Binding specificity of monoclonal antibodies towards the size variants of human growth hormone. *Molec. cell. Endocr.* **28**, 363–372.

Weeks, I., Kemp, H. A. and Woodhead, J. S. (1981). Two-site assay of human α-fetoprotein using ^{125}I-labelled monoclonal antibodies. *Biosci. Reports*, **1**, 785–791.

Weeks, I., Beheshti, I., McCapra, F., Campbell, A. K. and Woodhead, J. S. (1983). Acridinium esters as high specific activity labels in immunoassay. *Clin. Chem.* **29**, 1474–1479.

Weeks, I., Sturgess, M., Siddle, K., Jones, M. K. and Woodhead, J. S. (1984). A high-sensitivity immunochemiluminometric assay for human thyrotropin. *Clin. Endocr.* **20**, 489–495.

Woodhead, J. S., Addison, G. M. and Hales, C. N. (1974). The immunoradiometric assay and related techniques. *Br. Med. Bull.* **30**, 44–49.

CHAPTER 4

Particle immunoassays

H. van Hell, J. H. W. Leuvering and T. C. J. Gribnau
Diagnostic Research Laboratories,
Organon International BV,
Oss, The Netherlands

1. INTRODUCTION

The basis of every immunoassay is the reaction of an antibody with the corresponding antigen. If the concentrations of both reactants are sufficiently high and in the right proportion this reaction leads to a visible precipitate. However, the concentrations at which antigens and antibodies, which are of interest for diagnostic purposes, occur in body fluids are usually too low to produce a directly visible effect. Therefore, immunoassay development has concentrated on ways to detect the primary antigen–antibody reaction by means of secondary phenomena. Almost invariably this objective has been achieved by labelling the antigen or antibody with compounds or particles which allow easy or extremely sensitive detection.

During recent years, much attention has been focused on sophisticated methods like radioimmunoassay, enzyme immunoassay, fluoroimmunoassay and chemiluminescence immunoassay, which often allow the measurement of low levels of analyte. Such methods are often relatively complicated and require expensive equipment. Because of these developments, less attention has been given to earlier methods in which particles (such as erythrocytes, or polystyrene spheres) were used as labels for the antigen or antibody. Nevertheless, these methods have the advantage of simplicity of perform-ance, coupled to a sensitivity which is sufficient for many diagnostic applications. These characteristics account for the widespread use of the methods (e.g. for blood group typing, pregnancy and rheumatoid factor tests), and for our further attempts, and those of others, to improve the assay performance. In addition we have recently explored the use of other particles (gold sols and disperse dye sols) as labels in immunoassays, and novel shell/core particles have been reported for use in automated methods with a tubidimetric end-point (Litchfield *et al.*, 1984). In the present chapter we review the state of the art regarding particle immunoassays.

2. IMMUNOASSAYS USING ERYTHROCYTES

The agglutination of erythrocytes discovered by Landsteiner in 1901 was first used for blood group typing. Antibodies present in the serum of persons with blood group A react with antigens present on the erythrocytes of individuals with blood group B. When the reaction was performed on a glass slide the agglutination of the cells could be observed visually. This reaction, in which the reacting antigen is a natural part of the cell surface, was called haemagglutination (H). When an antigen attached to the cell acts as the reactant the reaction is called passive haemagglutination (PH). Reverse passive haemagglutination (RPH) is the reaction of an antibody bound to the cell surface with its antigen. Much better use of the sensitivity of the agglutination reaction of erythrocytes can be made by letting the cells sediment in test tubes or wells of microtitration plates. In the case of agglutination a diffuse pattern is formed in the bottom of the tube or well; in the absence of a reaction a ring or button pattern is observed (Fig. 1). In tests depending on H, PH or RPH a ring or button pattern therefore means a negative result; a diffuse pattern indicates a positive result.

Tests with red blood cells can, however, also be performed in the inhibition mode: antigen in the sample inhibits the reaction of antibody in solution with antigen attached to the erythrocytes. These types of tests are called passive haemagglutination inhibition (PHI) tests. Formation of a ring pattern (i.e. the absence of agglutination) in this case signals the presence of antigen, i.e. a positive result. To avoid confusion in the interpretation of results with HI and H tests we recently introduced a specially designed tube in a RPH test that produces a minus-like sedimentation pattern in the absence of agglutination, signifying a negative result (Fig. 1).

Fresh or stabilized erythrocytes can be used to bind antigens or antibodies. Stabilized erythrocytes are usually preferred since they can be stored for longer periods. Stabilization or fixation can be performed by treatment with formaldehyde, glutaraldehyde, pyruvic aldehyde or sulphosalicylic acid and numerous procedures and modifications have been described. The cell surface of erythrocytes allows the attachment of many different antigens, and those containing polysaccharides bind most strongly. Since the sensitivity of

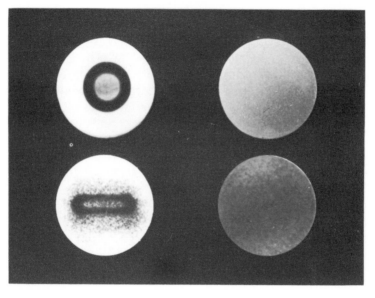

Result: Negative   Positive

Fig. 1. Sedimentation patterns of tube tests using erythrocytes

assays using erythrocytes depends on the amount of antigen or antibody bound per cell, the method used to adsorb or bind the protein to the cell surface is of great importance (Binns *et al.*, 1982).

There are three types of coating or sensitization of red blood cells for immunoassay: (i) the direct adsorption of antigen by the cells; (ii) the tanned cell technique, and (iii) covalent binding. The first method can be used for most proteins, but the sensitivity of the resultant cells can be much improved by previous tanning. The tanned cell technique (Boyden, 1951), in which fresh cells are treated with tannic acid, greatly enhances the amount of antigen that can be adsorbed, but also increases the tendency of the cells to agglutinate non-specifically. This tendency to self-agglutination can be reduced by the addition of normal serum. Boyden suggested that it was mainly the carbohydrate residues of molecules that bound to the tanned cell surface, although protein could also be adsorbed. Various methods have also been developed to bind antigen or antibody covalently to the cells, such as those using *bis*-diazotized benzidine (Pressman *et al.*, 1942), difluorodinitrobenzene (Ling, 1961), toluene 2,4-diisocyanate (Gyenes and Schon, 1964), carbodiimide (Johnson *et al.*, 1966), *bis*-diazotized *o*-dianisidine (Avrameas *et al.*, 1969) or indirectly via lectins (Sanderson, 1970). However, the continuous publication of modifications to these procedures suggest that while useful they are still not perfect. At present many alternative methods exist, but a common method of choice for every application is still lacking.

A modification of the haemagglutination principles described above is used in the viral haemagglutination inhibition tests. In these procedures use is made of viral receptors, which occur naturally on the surface of erythrocytes from many species. Antibodies against such viruses can be detected by their ability to inhibit the agglutination of such erythrocytes by the virus. Care should be taken to avoid interference of, for example, lipoproteins. These tests, for example, are widely used in the serology of rubella (Stewart et al., 1967). Other examples of large-scale applications of haemagglutination tests are: (i) hepatitis B surface antigen (HBsAg) and antibody (Vyas and Shulman, 1970; Cayzer et al., 1974; Schuurs and Kacaki, 1974), used in particular for the large-scale screening of blood donors, and (ii) haemagglutination inhibition tests for human chorionic gonadotrophin (hCG) in urine (Strausser, 1959; Wide and Gemzell, 1960; Polderman, 1962) to detect pregnancy [sensitivity: 1000 IU hCG (l urine)$^{-1}$]. The latter test, and one for human lutropin (hLH) (Schuurs and van Wijngaarden, 1969), were also used for the quantitative estimation of these hormones in urine. By applying reverse passive haemagglutination and two different monoclonal antibodies against hCG, one specific for the intact molecule and the other for the β-subunit, the sensitivity could be improved to 75 IU hCG (l urine)$^{-1}$ ($\sim$ 10 ng ml^{+1}). (van Hell and Helmich, 1984.)

These so-called tube tests are very popular because they possess a combination of very desirable properties. They are moderately to highly sensitive, very easy to perform and need no equipment other than a few pipettes and a settling rack. However, they are sensitive to vibrations that can disturb sedimentation patterns. A drawback of all assay systems using erythrocytes lies in their production. The red blood cell is a natural product and exhibits variable characteristics. Consequently, it is still difficult to manufacture tests with defined properties over long periods of time.

3. IMMUNOASSAYS USING LATEX PARTICLES

These assays are based on the agglutination of antigen- or antibody-coated polystyrene (latex) spheres due to analyte added to the aqueous suspension of particles. Since the success of assay systems based on erythrocytes, investigators have been looking for other particles with more constant properties. Singer and Plotz in 1956 were the first to use a suspension of polystyrene particles coated with immunoglobulins to detect rheumatoid factor (RF). The reaction was carried out in a test tube and the agglutination of the particles could be observed with the naked eye.

Following this discovery the development of similar assays proceeded in two directions: the first led to the further perfection of tests that could be read by the naked eye, while the second aimed at the development of sophisticated equipment to measure the agglutination in the initial phase of the process. For the visual detection a number of tube tests were developed for RF (Singer and Plotz, 1956), anti-DNA antibodies (Christian *et al.*, 1958), hCG (Robbins *et al.*, 1962), and *Brucella* antigen and antiserum (Fleck and Evenchik, 1962). The real advantage of this new particle, however, only became apparent when the agglutination was allowed to develop on a slide. Thus a drop of reagent, containing antigen- or antibody-coated latex in suspension was mixed on a flat surface (a slide) with a drop of sample (urine, serum or plasma). After gentle rocking of the slide for 2 or 3 min the agglutination pattern could be read with the naked eye. These latex tests became very popular in serology, and as pregnancy tests, although they were generally somewhat less sensitive than the tube tests using erythrocytes.

Recently, it has been shown that by using direct agglutination, with smaller particles and monoclonal antibodies, the sensitivity of latex slide tests for hCG can be increased to about 250–500 IU ($\sim$25–50 μg) hCG (1 urine)$^{-1}$. This improvement illustrates that further possibilities exist, especially if other types of latex particles and covalent binding are explored. However, the formation of a visible agglutination in such a short time still requires a relatively high concentration of the substance to be measured, which explains the lower sensitivity of slide tests as compared with sophisticated immunotests such as radioimmunoassay (RIA) and enzyme immunoassay (EIA). Obviously the sensitivity of latex tests could be greatly improved if a more early phase of the agglutination, invisible to the naked eye, could be detected.

The technique of quasi-elastic light-scattering spectroscopy (Benedek, 1969) provides a sensitive, quantitative and accurate method. It measures the average diffusion constant of the particles, which is a function of their size. With this technique a sensitivity of 10–20 μg antibody l^{-1} could be realised (Cohen and Benedek, 1975). Since a visible agglutinate with the same reagents required a concentration of 2–5 mg l^{-1}, this technique yielded a 100-fold increase in sensitivity. A minimum concentration in urine of 16 IU hCG l^{-1} could be detected (von Schulthess *et al.*, 1976). By using angular anisotropy measurement the sensitivity could be further improved to 2 IU hCG (1 urine)$^{-1}$ (von Schulthess *et al.*, 1980). However, when this technique was used for measurements in serum, non-specific agglutination and inhibitory effects were observed. New developments in this area became possible by the introduction of particle counting immunoassay (PACIA) (Cambiaso *et al.*, 1977). This technique involves the measurement of the number of residual non-agglutinated particles by means of equipment designed to count blood cells. Using the IgG fractions of goat antisera against human placental lactogen (hPL) and α-fetoprotein (AFP) to coat latex particles, threshold sensitivities of 10 μg (1 buffer)$^{-1}$ could be reached for these proteins. However, to suppress serum interference the samples had to be treated with dithiothreitol and subsequently diluted, which reduced the sensitivity to 100 $\mu g \ l^{-1}$. The use of F (ab')$_2$ fragments to coat latex particles and a high ionic strength in the reaction medium considerably reduced the interference from serum. In this way the dose range for AFP could be improved to 10–500 μg (l serum)$^{-1}$ (Collet-Cassart et al., 1981).

The combined use of F (ab')$_2$ fragments, slightly dissociating conditions by a chaotropic agent, such as ammonium thiocyanate, and chelation of bivalent cations by EDTA enabled ferritin to be detected at a lower limit of 13 μg (l serum)$^{-1}$ (Limet et al., 1982). The assay of C-reactive protein in serum, cord serum and cerebrospinal fluid was reported recently (Collet-Cassart et al., 1983). Sera were diluted 10 times and cerebrospinal fluid twice with an assay having a range extending from 1 to 100 $\mu g \ l^{-1}$. PACIA obviously has several advantages such as: (i) no separation step is required; (ii) the incubation times are short, and (iii) the process is fully automated. A disadvantage is the need to use large and expensive equipment and the sensitivity obtained does not completely match that of radioimmunoassay and enzyme immunoassay.

4. IMMUNOASSAYS USING INORGANIC COLLOIDAL PARTICLES

As was shown in our laboratories, aqueous dispersions of inorganic colloidal particles (sols) possess a number of properties which render them suitable for use as labels in immunoassays. In accordance with the nomenclature of RIA and EIA, assays based on the use of sol particles as a label are named sol particle immunoassay (SPIA). Although most of the work described here concerns colloidal gold particles, other types of colloidal particles may be used as well.

4.1. Homogeneous (non-separation) SPIAs

Homogeneous SPIA takes advantage of two important properties of gold sols, viz. their typical red colour, which is not affected by the adsorption of antibodies (Ab) to the particles, and the considerable change of the light absorption spectrum, and hence the colour, accompanying the aggregation. This change in the light absorption spectrum is reflected by a decrease of the absorbance at 540 nm (A_{540nm}). The aggregation of antibody-coated, 50 nm gold particles (Au_{50}–Ab) by an immunochemically polyvalent antigen is named agglutination, and immunoassays based on this process are called agglutination SPIAs. These assays are extremely easy to perform. Aliquots of a buffered dispersion of Au_{50}–Ab and the (diluted) sample or standard solution are pipetted into a reaction vessel and mixed. After a fixed incubation period (e.g. 0.5–2 h) the A_{540nm} of the reaction mixture is measured, or the colour is assessed visually. If the antigen is present at a suitable concentration, Au_{50}–Ab is agglutinated, which results in a lower value of A_{540nm}, or, when inspected visually, by a colour change. If the antigen is absent, or the concentration is too low the A_{540nm} remains at its initial level, and the colour of the reaction mixture does not change (Leuvering et al., 1981). A low degree of agglutination produces a colour shift from red towards purple or blue, while the formation of large aggregates results in a grey colour. After sedimentation of the aggregated particles the supernatant eventually becomes colourless.

The latter property allowed the development of a screening test for the presence of hCG in urine, the result of which could be assessed by visual inspection. A considerable improvement of the specificity of this test was achieved by replacing the anti-hCG from rabbit antisera by mouse monoclonal anti-hCG. The main advantage of monoclonal anti-hCG is the possibility of selecting clones that produce antibodies which have the optimum combination of properties such as affinity, a low level of cross-reaction with hLH and non-specific interactions with sample components. This development resulted in a test for pregnancy, which is also suitable for use by a lay person. The test is able to detect about 450 IU hCG (l urine)$^{-1}$, which corresponds to about 2.1 nmol l^{-1}. If a colorimeter is used to measure the A_{540nm} of the reaction mixture the sensitivity of the test is 280 IU hCG l^{-1}, corresponding to about 1.3 nmol l^{-1} (Leuvering et al., 1983a).

Recent work using new combinations of monoclonal anti-hCG antibodies shows that the sensitivity of the colorimetric agglutination SPIA for hCG in urine can be improved by at least a factor of 3 (Fig. 2). Consequently a detection limit of 100 IU l^{-1} seems possible. Since haptens, e.g. steroids and drugs, are immunochemically monovalent, they cannot be detected by a direct agglutination assay. However, immunochemically multivalent hapten complexes, consisting of bovine serum albumin (BSA) molecules to which several hapten molecules per BSA molecule (h-BSA) have been coupled, are able to agglutinate anti-hapten (anti-h)-coated gold particles [Au_{50}–(anti-h)]. The agglutination of Au_{50}–(anti-h) can be inhibited by hapten molecules from the sample or the standard solution. The test procedure consists of three pipetting steps: (i) the sample or standard solution; (ii) the buffered Au_{50}–(anti-h), and (iii) the buffer containing a fixed amount of h-BSA to initiate the agglutination reaction. After a fixed incubation period the absorbance of the reaction mixture is measured by a colorimeter. This type of assay was used to measure the concentration of oestrogens in urine or serum samples (Leuvering et al., 1983b). After extraction and dilution with buffer, oestrogen concentrations in the range of 2–10 μg l^{-1} (7–35 μmol l^{-1}) were measured, which illustrates that this method is probably suitable for the assay of other haptens.

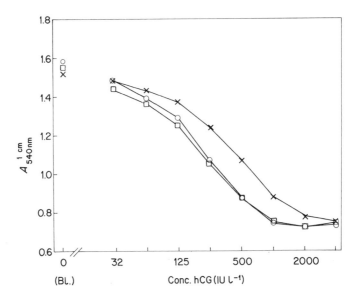

Fig. 2. Agglutination SPIA for hCG in urine, using monoclonal antibodies against the hormone. Each curve represents the result with a different combination of antibodies adsorbed to the well and to the gold sol. Procedure: add 40 μl of sample and 160 μl of buffered Au_{50}–(anti hCG) to each well of a microtitration plate, mix by vibration, and incubate for 0.5 h at room temperature; measure absorbance, □–□, ○–○ and x–x represent different combinations of monoclonal antibodies

4.2. Heterogeneous (separation) SPIAs

The sandwich and the sandwich inhibition SPIA are examples of a group of heterogeneous assays. In the sandwich SPIA an aliquot of the sample or standard solution is incubated with an antibody-coated polystyrene well (PS–Ab) of a microtitration plate. The antigen to be assayed is bound to PS–Ab, after which the well is washed and incubated with a fixed (excess) amount of Au_{50}–Ab. During the latter incubation step the antigen molecules bound to PS–Ab also bind Au_{50}–Ab. The excess amount of Au_{50}–Ab can be removed and the Au_{50}–Ab bound to the wall of the well can be redispersed by adding a fixed aliquot of a base or an acid which dissociates the immune complexes. Depending on the sensitivity required, various methods can be used to detect or quantitate the redispersed bound fraction of Au_{50}–Ab. A detection limit of about 170 pmol l^{-1} was obtained by visual inspection of the redispersed bound fraction of Au_{50}–Ab (Leuvering et al., 1980). If colorimetry is used after overnight incubation to quantitate this fraction the detection limit for hCG is about 1 IU l^{-1} (5 pmol) (see, for example, Fig. 3). With a total incubation time of 4 h the detection limit is about 4 IU l^{-1}. Using

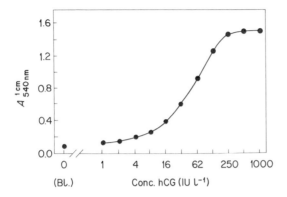

Fig. 3. Sandwich SPIA for hCG in urine using rabbit anti-hCG. Procedure: add 100 μl of sample to an anti-hCG coated well of a microtitration plate and incubate for 2 h at 37 °C; aspirate and wash twice using 300 μl of buffer, add 100 μl of a buffered Au_{50}–(anti-hCG) dispersion and incubate for 16 h at 37 °C, aspirate and wash four times. Add 110 μl of 0.1 mol l^{-1} NaOH to the wells, homogenize the dispersion by vibration and measure the absorbance

atomic absorption spectrophotometry (AAS) for detection, concentrations as low as 4 mIU l^{-1} (about 20 fmol l^{-1}) were measured in buffer (Leuvering, 1984a). Another procedure for the detection of antigen in the sample by sandwich SPIA is direct inspection of the colour of the wall of the well after removal of the excess AU_{50}–Ab. The presence of antigen is accompanied by a red or pink colour of the wall, which remains colourless in the absence of the analyte. Since in the colorimetric SPIA a considerable amount of the added Au_{50}–Ab can be bound, it is also possible to construct a dose–response curve by measuring the absorbance of the free fraction of Au_{50}–Ab (Leuvering et al., 1983c). Simultaneous measurement of the concentration of two non-cross-reacting antigens, e.g. hCG and human placental lactogen (hPL), in the same aliquot was possible using polystyrene wells coated with a mixture of anti-hPL and anti-hCG, a mixture of Au_{50}–(anti-hCG) and Ag_{50}–(anti-hPL) and measurement of the concentration of Au and Ag in the redispersed bound fractions of Au_{50}–(anti-hCG) and Ag_{50}–(anti-hPL) by AAS (Leuvering et al., 1980). The effects of the assay procedure and reagent properties on the dose–response curve and matrix interference are described by Leuvering et al. (1983c).

Haptens cannot be assayed by a sandwich SPIA for the same reasons as mentioned for the agglutination SPIA. However, an immunochemically multivalent h-BSA conjugate can be used in a sandwich SPIA. A fixed suitable amount of h-BSA will result in a constant and sufficiently high level of A_{540nm} for the redispersed bound fraction of Au_{50}–(anti-h). The binding of h-BSA to PS–(anti-h) can be inhibited by free hapten molecules. A decrease in the amount of h-BSA bound to PS–(anti-h) is reflected by a decrease in the fraction of Au_{50}–(anti-h) bound to PS–(anti-h)–h-BSA. This type of SPIA, the sandwich inhibition SPIA, is in principle suitable to measure the concentration of haptens such as testosterone (Leuvering, 1984b). Although the present system requires improvement to obtain an operational assay, the present test procedure and reagents resulted in a detection limit of 1.7 μg of testosterone per litre in buffer using colorimetry for detection.

5. DISPERSE DYE IMMUNOASSAY (DIA)

The application of hydrophobic, colloidal dye particles as labels in immunoassays has been described (Gribnau et al., 1982, 1983). These particles can be used as labels in two essentially different ways: (i) in an agglutination assay where the immunoreaction results in the formation of dye particle aggregates which can be detected visually or optically, or (ii) in a sandwich assay, taking advantage of the colour properties of the dye particles, which can be detected directly, or more particularly after their dissolution into an organic solvent. Dye sol particles were used in agglutination assays as previously described (Gribnau et al., 1982). Further experimental evaluation indicated, however, that gold sol particles were to be preferred in this type of assay. This finding is due to the considerably higher specific density of gold as compared to organic dyes, and to the fact that the aggregation of gold sol particles yields a distinct change in colour.

The characteristic properties of colloidal dye particles may be used to advantage, however, by applying them as labels in sandwich-type immunoassays (Fig. 4). The particular advantage lies in the amplification of the detection signal (absorbance) achieved by the final dissolution of the dye particles, yielding a monomolecular dye solution. The advantage of dye sol labelling over molecular dye labelling (by covalent coupling of separate dye molecules to antibodies) is obvious. The number of dye molecules per immunocomplex is considerably (at least 1000 times) higher in the former

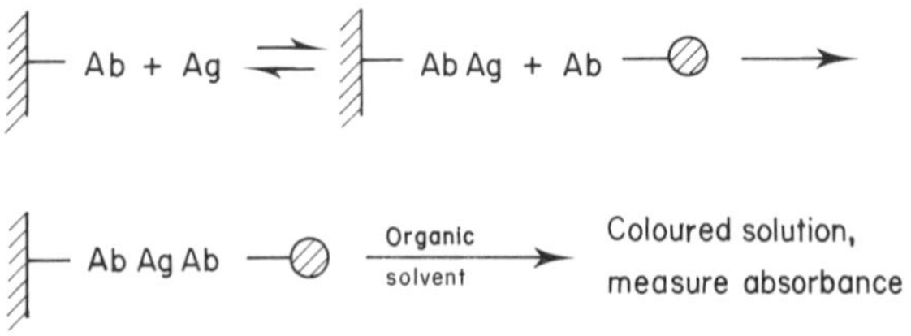

Fig. 4. Reaction principle of a sandwich disperse dye immunoassay. Hatched rule indicates solid phase (microtitration plate); hatched circles indicate dye sol particles; Ab, antibody; Ag, antigen from sample

case. Model calculations have been described previously (Gribnau *et al.*, 1982). In colorimetric sandwich-type immunoassays, dye particle labels have an advantage over gold sols due to the substantially higher molar absorbances (ϵ) of the organic dyes. For example: gold sol, particle size ~50 nm, produces values for ϵ of 3000–4000 1 mol^{-1} cm^{-1} (J.H.W. Leuvering, personal communication); disperse dyes, however, have ϵ values of 5000–80000 1 mol^{-1} cm^{-1} (Venkataraman, 1977).

Labelled reagents which are chemically well defined, stable and non-radioactive can be prepared easily from a wide range of commercially available disperse dyes. The labelling of antibodies is performed by simple physical adsorption, and several detection methods can be used to detect the end-point of the immunoassay, e.g. visual observation, colorimetry, fluorometry and (carbon rod) atomic absorption spectrophotometry (in the case of metal-complex dyes). Experimental aspects, generally important for the successful development of labelled sandwich immunoassays, equally apply to DIA: e.g. the type of solid phase (microtitration plate), the quality of the antibodies (specificity, affinity, source, poly/monoclonal) and general assay conditions (incubation periods, temperature, pH, concentration of reagents, sample interference). Some essential features of DIA are the properties of the dyes, i.e. particle size, distribution and shape; solubility in appropriate organic solvents; value of the molar absorbance; colloid-chemical stability of the dye sol; conditions for adsorptive antibody immobilization; binding capacity of the dye particles for IgG; and stability of the adsorptive dye particle–antibody bond.

Commercially available 'disperse dyes' (Straley, 1970) were taken as starting material for the preparation of the dye sols. These are defined according to the Colour Index as: 'A class of substantially water-insoluble dyes originally introduced for dyeing cellulose acetate, and usually applied from fine aqueous suspensions; now also widely used for the colouration of all hydrophobic synthetic fibres' (Blackshaw and Brightman 1961). The dye sols were prepared by centrifugal fractionation of the aqueous dispersions. The labelling of antibodies was performed by their adsorptive immobilization on the dye particles, followed by a secondary coating with bovine serum albumin, yielding finally the so-called 'conjugates'. The conjugates are stable for at least 15 months (at $-20\,°C$ or $4\,°C$), provided that they are stored in the lyophilized state. Aqueous conjugates should be used within 6 days of preparation.

Sandwich immunoassays were performed using antibody-coated, poly-styrene microtitration plates. The sample is incubated for 30 min at 37 °C. The conjugate is added and the mixture incubated for 2 h at 37 °C. The bound dye label is dissolved into an organic solvent and the absorbance read in a spectrophometer. All experimental procedures, materials and reagents have been described in detail (Gribnau *et al.*, 1983; recent investigations showed dimethyl sulphoxide to be a better alternative to ℓ-propanol).

Disperse dyes suitable for conjugate preparation can be found only by screening. The particular selection may also depend on the type of antibody preparation that is used. Good representatives are Foron ® Brilliant Blue SR (Sandoz), Terasil ® Brilliant Flavin 8GFF (Ciba-Geigy), Palanil® Luminous Red G and Palanil® Yellow 3GE (BASF). Finally, prepared dye sols with a particle size distribution corresponding to a modal effective diameter of ~200 nm (or ~300 nm median; Fischer, 1950) yielded optimal conjugates. The shape of the particles should be as spherical as possible. The pH during conjugate preparation was rather critical when mouse monoclonal antibodies were used, but was of minor importance in the case of polyclonal rabbit antibodies; the optimal pH was also dye dependent. The type of dye and antibody also determined the value of the pH to be applied during conjugate incubation in order to achieve maximum response and a minimum blank.

The assay protocol for DIA also depends upon the type of antibody used (cf. Fig. 4). Separate, sequential incubation of sample and conjugate is necessary in the case of polyclonal antibodies ('DIA-I'). Sample and conjugate can be incubated simultaneously when the conjugate is based on monoclonal antibodies ('DIA-II'), yielding a simplified assay procedure. In summary:

DIA-I	DIA-II
Add sample	
Incubate, 0.5 h; 37 °C	
Aspirate and wash	
Add conjugate	Add conjugate and sample
Incubate, 2 h; 37 °C	Incubate, 2.5 h; 37 °C
Aspirate and wash	Aspirate and wash
Add organic solvent	Add organic solvent
Determine absorbance	Determine absorbance

The results of both assay protocols for the hCG/anti-hCG system, using hCG-containing samples in buffer, urine (pooled), serum (pooled) and diluted serum randomized over 12 microtitration plates, are given in Figs. 5 and 6. The detection limit (DL) for hCG in buffer was about 2 IU l^{-1} in 'DIA-I' (DL is defined as the hCG concentration yielding a response equal to blank + 3 × standard deviation). Serum interference clearly impairs the results, particularly in the case of 'DIA-II'. There is also a considerable difference in response when different sera, spiked with the same concentration of hCG, are used instead of pooled serum (Fig. 7). The possible reduction of these effects by using $F(ab')_2$ fragments instead of total IgG is being investigated.

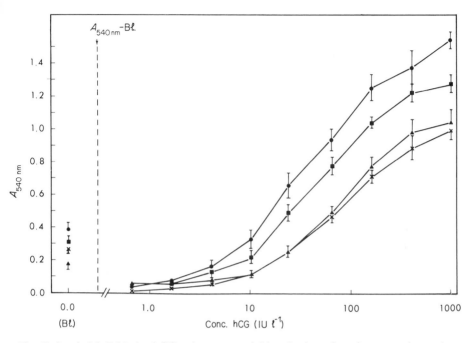

Fig. 5. Sandwich DIA for hCG using sequential incubation of conjugate and sample ('DIA-I'). Plate wells are coated with rabbit anti-hCG; conjugate is mouse monoclonal anti-hCG/Palanil [®] Luminous Red G. All points represent the mean value for six replicate sample. ●–●, buffer; ▲–▲, urine; x–x, serum; ■–■, 10% v/v serum. Error bars are standard errors.

Most of the exploratory and developmental investigations have been performed using hCG/anti-hCG as a model system. Sandwich DIAs were also used, however, for the determination of hPL, human prolactin and testosterone (Gribnau *et al.*, 1982). In the latter case a sandwich inhibition assay was used as described for oestriol (Schuurs *et al.*, 1982; Leuvering, 1984b). The determination of tumour markers, for example α-fetoprotein (AFP), is being investigated, using pooled human sera spiked with the analyte. A detection limit of 5 μg l^{-1} can be obtained. This system requires further optimization.

An attractive feature of the sandwich DIA is that it allows two different antigens to be determined simultaneously, using the corresponding antibodies labelled with differently coloured dye particles, which are clearly distinguishable spectrophotometrically. Blue and yellow chromophores, yielding various shades of green upon subtractive colour mixing (Schultze, 1975; Simon, 1980), are particularly suitable for this application. The high sensitivity of the human eye for various shades of green (Hardy, 1936; Rösch, 1964) could

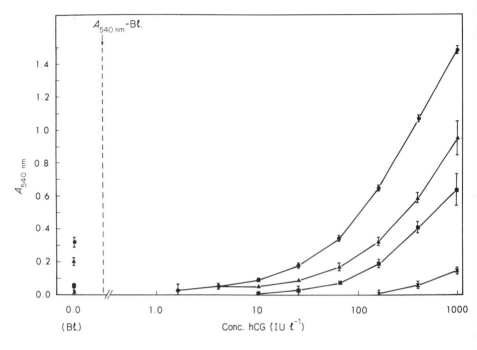

Fig. 6. Sandwich DIA for hCG with the simultaneous incubation of conjugate and sample ('DIA–II'). Conditions and symbols as in Fig. 5

possibly enable the development of eye-reading tests for the qualitative determination of antigen ratios. An example of the simultaneous determination of hCG and hPL is given in Fig. 8 (Gribnau *et al.*, 1982).

6. DISCUSSION

The present applications of particle immunoassays, in particular the systems using erythrocytes and latex particles, are in the field of eye reading tests. In this area they have obtained a dominant position because of their ease of operation. Their sensitivities are good enough for use as screening tests (e.g. hepatitis, rubella, pregnancy) and in some cases are adequate for quantitative methods. In particular the tests using erythrocytes are suitable for the latter application since their sedimentation patterns facilitate statistical evaluation. In the last decade, however, enzyme immunoassay (EIA) has made progress in this field of application, mainly because this technique generally has a higher sensitivity and makes it possible to diminish interference from urine or serum by separation of the antibody bound and free fractions. In assays using

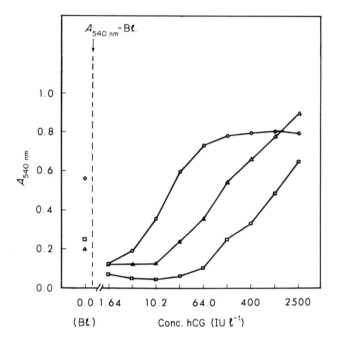

Fig. 7. Sandwich DIA for hCG with the simultaneous incubation of conjugate and sample ('DIA–II'): effect of serum interference. Plate wells coated with mouse monoclonal anti-hCG; the conjugate is mouse monoclonal anti-hCG/Palanil ® Luminous Red G (different types of monoclonal anti-hCG were used for plate well and conjugate). O–O, buffer; □–□, normal human serum 8433/82–312; △–△, normal human serum 8307/82–19

erythrocytes, or latex particles, only one incubation step is used, and interfering factors from the sample are present in the same solution where the final assay response is read. These interfering factors can therefore affect both the primary reaction between antibody and antigen and the final reaction, agglutination and/or sedimentation of the particles). In EIAs only the antibody–antigen reaction can be affected; the final enzyme reaction is protected from interference by the separation of the antibody bound fraction.

Recent developments, summarized for hCG-tests in Table 1, have shown that improvements and innovations in the field of particle immunoassays are still possible. For example, the introduction of monoclonal antibodies in reverse agglutination tests led to a considerable improvement in sensitivity (i.e. to 75 IU hCG l^{-1} for tests using erythrocytes and to 250 IU hCG l^{-1} for tests depending on latex particles). The replacement of variable antisera by these new reagents also improved the reproducibility of manufactured tests.

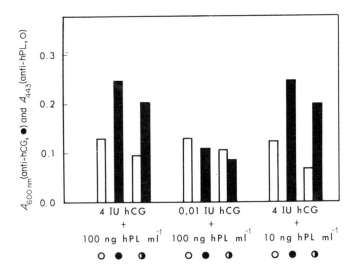

Fig. 8. Simultaneous determination of hCG and hPL by sandwich DIA using a 1:1 mixture (○) of rabbit anti-hCG/Resolin ® Brilliant Blue RRL (●) and rabbit anti-hPL/Palanil ® Yellow 3G (○); the response of the single conjugates is also given. [Reproduced by permission of Elsevier Scientific Publishing Company from Gribnau *et al.* (1982).]

Developments in the field of latex particle assays have also taken place: (i) in the construction of sophisticated equipment to measure agglutination in the initial phases of the process, which has increased the sensitivity of the method; and (ii) in finding measures to reduce the effect of interfering substances in biological samples, which again improved the practical sensitivity.

A recent innovation was the application of colloidal gold particles. The use of this particle with a diameter of approximately 50 nm, coated with antibody, as an immunoreagent, considerably improved the sensitivity of particle immunoassays. It also introduced an entirely new method for reading the end-point of the reaction of a homogeneous SPIA: the reduction of the specific absorbance of gold sols brought about by agglutination can be read by eye (yes/no tests) and by a spectrophotometer (quantitative tests). A practical advantage of the homogeneous SPIA is that after mixing reagent and sample it needs neither the rocking action of the latex slide test nor the disturbance-free settling period of the erythrocyte test. It is probably the easiest test to perform. By measuring the decrease of the absorbance at 540 nm, a quantitative test for hCG can be obtained with a sensitivity of 100 IU (l urine)$^{-1}$. Sample interference is a problem in the agglutination SPIA, as in other homogeneous assays. Applied in a sandwich-type assay, a detection

Table 1. Particle immunoassay systems for hCG

Particle	Method	Sensitivity	Remarks
Erythrocyte	Reverse passive haemagglutination	75 IU (l urine)$^{-1}$	Simple procedure; assay time 2 h
Latex	Agglutination, eye-reading	250 IU (l urine)$^{-1}$	Simple procedure; assay time 3 min
Latex	Agglutination, instrument reading	2 IU (l urine)$^{-1}$	Instrumentation necessary; complicated; expensive
Gold particle	Agglutination, eye-reading	450 IU (l urine)$^{-1}$	Simple procedure; assay time 0.5 h
Gold particle	Agglutination, colorimeter	100 IU (l urine)$^{-1}$	Simple instrumentation; assay time 0.5 h
Gold particle	sandwich, colorimeter	4 IU (l buffer)$^{-1}$	Simple instrumentation; assay time 4 h
Gold particle	Sandwich carbon rod atomic absorption spectrophotometry (CRAAS)	4 mIU (l buffer)$^{-1}$	Expensive instrumentation; overnight incubation
Disperse dye Palanil® Luminous Red G	Sandwich colorimeter	3.5 IU (l urine)$^{-1}$	Simple instrumentation; assay time 3 h

limit of 1 IU hCG per litre of buffer (5 pmol l^{-1}) can be reached when colorimetry is used. Using atomic absorption spectrophotometry a concentration of hCG in buffer of 4 mIU l^{-1} (20 fmol l^{-1}) can be measured.

A new principle was introduced in particle immunoassay when disperse dyes were used for the preparation of conjugates. The high sensitivity of DIA is accomplished by dissolving the dye particle into an organic solvent in the final step of the assay. Every molecule of the particle makes its contribution to the absorbance measured in the solution. A sensitivity similar to or better than that reached with the sandwich SPIA (4 h incubation) using colorimetry can be obtained. However, assays using different serum samples clearly showed that as with SPIA serum interference is reducing the practical sensitivity of this assay type. Therefore it seems that in assays using latex or gold sols or disperse dyes, this problem must be solved before the sensitivity can be improved further.

In conclusion, we expect the agglutination SPIA to be the most promising new technique in the field of yes/no tests. The process which most clearly requires further improvement in the preparation of both sensitized erythrocytes and latex particles is the reproducible binding of antibody or antigen to the particle. Binding methods that prevent leakage of antibody or antigen from the particles and which do not alter the immunochemical activity of the substance bound may improve the sensitivity and reproducibility of these types of immunoassays.

ACKNOWLEDGEMENTS

The authors are grateful to the Photography Group of Organon SDG for the figures and to Miss F. Veerkamp and Mrs M. Gerlach for typing the manuscript.

REFERENCES

Avrameas, S., Taudou, B. and Chuilon, S. (1969). Glutaraldehyde, cyanuric chloride and tetraazotized o-dianisidine as coupling reagents in the passive hemagglutination test. *Immunochemistry* **6**, 67–76.

Benedek, G. B. (1969). *Polarization, Matter and Radiation*, Presses Universitaire de France, Paris, pp.49–84.

Binns, R. M., Licence, S. T., Gurner, B. W. and Coombs, R. R. A. (1982). Factors which govern the sensitivity of direct and indirect rosetting reactions and reverse passive haemagglutination in the identification of cell surface and free macromolecules. *Immunology* **47**, 717–727.

Blackshaw, H. and Brightman, R. (1961). *Dictionary of Dyeing and Textile Printing*, George Newnes Ltd, London, p.62.

Boyden, S. V. (1951). The adsorption of protein on erythrocytes treated with tannic acid and subsequent hemagglutination by antiprotein sera. *J. exp. Med.* **93**, 107–120.

Cambiaso, C. L., Leek, A. E., de Steenwinkel, F., Billen, J. and Masson, P. L. (1977). Particle counting immunoassay (PACIA). I. A general method for the determination of antibodies, antigens and haptens. *Immunol Methods* **18**, 33–44.

Cayzer, I., Dane, D. S., Cameron, C. H. and Denning, J. V. (1974). A rapid haemagglutination test for hepatitis-B antigen. *Lancet*, **7**, 947–949.

Christian, C. L., Bryan, R. M. and Larson, D. L. (1958) Latex agglutination test for disseminated lupus erythematosus. *Proc. Soc. exp. Biol. Med.* **98**, 820–823.

Cohen, R. J. and Benedek, G. B. (1975). Immunoassay by light scattering spectroscopy. *Immunochemistry* **12**, 349–351.

Collet-Cassart, D., Magnusson, C. G. M., Ratcliffe, J. G., Cambiaso, C. L. and Masson, P. L. (1981). Automated particle-counting immunoassay for alphafetoprotein. *Clin. Chem.* **27**, 64–67.

Collet-Cassart, D., Mareschal, J. C., Sindic, C. J. M., Tomassi, T. P. and Masson, P. L. (1983). Automated particle counting immunoassay of C-reactive protein. Application to serum, cord serum and cerebrospinal fluid. *Clin. Chem.* **29**, 1127–1131.

Fischer, E. K. (1950). *Colloidal Dispersions*, John Wiley, London, pp. 3–15.

Fleck, L. and Evenchik, Z. (1962). Latex agglutination test with *Brucella* antigen and antiserum. *Nature, Lond.* **194**, 548–550.

Gribnau, T., Roeles, R., Biezen, J. van der, Leuvering, J. and Schuurs, A. (1982). The application of colloidal dye particles as label in immunoassays: disperse(d) dye immunoassay ('DIA'). In *Affinity Chromatography and Related Techniques* Series,

Vol. 9, (T. C. J. Gribnau, J. Visser and R. J. F. Nivard, eds), Analytical Chemistry Symposia, Elsevier, Amsterdam, pp. 411–424.

Gribnau, T., Sommeren, A. van and Dinther, F. van (1983). DIA–disperse dye immunoassay. In *Affinity Chromatography and Biological Recognition* (I. M. Chaiken, M. Wilchek and I. Parikh, eds), Academic Press, New York, pp. 375–380.

Gyenes, L. and Schon, A. H. (1964). The use of toluene 2,4-diisocyanate as a coupling agent in the passive hemagglutination rection. *Immunochemistry* 1, 43–48.

Hardy, A. C. (1936). *Handbook of Colorimetry*, Massachusetts Institute of Technology Press, Cambridge, Mass., USA, p. 9.

van Hell, H. and Helmich, J. (1984). Pregnancy testing: Applications of monoclonal technology. *Biotechnology Laboratory* 2, 22–33.

Johnson, H. M., Brenner, K. and Hall, H. E. (1966). The use of a water soluble carbodiimide as a coupling reagent in the passive hemagglutination test. *J. Immunol.* 97, 791–1796.

Leuvering, J. H. W. (1984a). Dose–response curves for HCG in buffer obtained in a sandwich SPIA using atomic absorption spectrophotometry for measuring the redispersed bound Au–(anti HCG) fraction. In thesis entitled 'Sol particle immunoassay (SPIA): the use of antibody coated particles as labelled antibodies in various types of immunoassay'.

Leuvering, J. H. W. (1984b). A sandwich inhibition sol particle immunoassay for haptens using testosterone as an example; a preliminary study. In thesis entitled 'Sol particle immunoassay (SPIA): the use of antibody coated particles as labelled antibodies in various types of immunoassay'.

Leuvering, J. H. W., Thal, P. J. H. M., Waart, M. van der, and Schuurs, A. H. W. M. (1980). Sol particle immunoassay (SPIA). *J. Immunoassay* 1, 77–91.

Leuvering, J. H. W., Thal, P. J. H. M., Waart, M. van der and Schuurs, A. H. W. M. (1981). A sol particle agglutination assay for human chorionic gonadotrophin. *J. Immunol. Meth.* 45, 183–194.

Leuvering, J. H. W., Goverde, B. C., Thal, P. J. H. M. and Schuurs, A. H. W. M. (1983a). A homogeneous sol particle immunoassay for human chorionic gonadotrophin using monoclonal antibodies. *J. Immunol. Meth.* 60, 9–23.

Leuvering, J. H. W., Thal, P. J. H. M., White, D. D. and Schuurs, A. H. W. M. (1983b). A homogeneous sol particle immunoassay for total oestrogens in urine and serum samples. *J. Immunol. Meth.* 62, 163–174.

Leuvering, J. H. W., Thal, P. J. H. M. and Schuurs, A. H. W. M. (1983c). Optimization of a sandwich sol particle immunoassay for human chorionic gonadotrophin. *J. Immunol. Meth.*, 62, 175–184.

Limet, J. N., Collet-Cassart, D. and Magnusson, C. G. M. (1982). Particle counting immunoassay (PACIA) of ferritin. *J. clin. Chem clin. Biochem.* 20, 141–146.

Ling, N. R. (1961). The coupling of protein antigens to erythrocytes with difluorodinitrobenzene. *Immunology* 4, 49–54.

Litchfield, W. J., Craig, A. R., Frey, W. A., Leflar, C. C., Looney, C. E. and Luddy, M. A. (1984). Novel shell/core particles for automated turbidimetric immunoassays. *Clin. Chem.* 30, 1489–1493.

Polderman, J. (1962). Een eenvoudige immunologische zwangerschaps reactie. *Pharm. Weekblad* 97, 529–546.

Pressman, D., Campbell, D. H. and Pauling, L. (1942). The agglutination of intact azoerythrocytes by antisera homologous to the attached groups. *J. Immunol.* 44, 101–105.

Robbins, J. L., Hill, G. A., Carle, B. N., Carlquist, J. H. and Marcus, C. (1962). Latex agglutination reactions between human chorionic gonadotropin and rabbit antibody. *Proc. Soc. exp. Biol. Med.* **109**, 321–325.

Rösch, S. (1964). Farbenlehre auf die Mathematik angewandt. *Palette*, **15**, 22.

Sanderson, C. J. (1970). Lectins and lipopolysaccharides as linking agents for the red cell linked antigen test. *Immunology* **18**, 353–360.

Schulthess, K. G. von, Cohen, R. J. and Benedek, G. B. (1976). Laser light scattering spectroscopic immunoassay in the agglutination inhibition mode for human chorionic gonadotropin (hCG) and human luteinizing hormone (hLH). *Immunochemistry* **13**, 963–966.

Schulthess, K. G. von, Giglio, M., Cannel, D. S. and Benedek, G. B. (1980). Detection of agglutination reactions using anisotropic light scattering: An immunoassay of high sensitivity. *Molec. Immunol.* **17**, 81–92.

Schultze, W. (1975). *Farbenlehre und Farbenmessung*, Springer, Berlin, p. 49.

Schuurs, A. H. W. M., Gribnau, T. C. J. and Leuvering, J. H. W. (1982). Use of immobilized reagents in immunoassay. In *Affinity Chromatography and Related Techniques* (T. C. J. Gribnau, J. Visser and R. J. F. Nivard, eds), Analytical Chemistry Symposia Series, Vol. 9, Elsevier, Amsterdam, pp. 343–356.

Schuurs, A. and Kacaki, J. (1974). Der umgekehrte Hämagglutinationstest für Hepatitis B-Antigen. In *Forschungsergebnisse der Transfusionsmedizin und Immunhaematologie* (M. Matthes and V. Nagel, eds), Medicus, Berlin, pp. 645–652.

Schuurs, A. H. W. M. and Wijngaarden, C. J. van (1969). A modified haemagglutination inhibition test and its application for the estimation of human luteinizing hormone in unconcentrated urine. *Acta Endocr., Copenh.* Suppl. 141, 13–31.

Simon, F. T. (1980). Color order. In *Color Measurement, Optical Radiation Measurements* Vol. 2, (F. Grumm and C. J. Bartleson, eds), Academic Press, New York, pp. 175–180, 182–186.

Singer, J. M. and Plotz, C. M. (1956). The latex fixation test. *Am. J. Med.* **21**, 888–892.

Stewart, G. L., Parkman, P. D., Hopps, H. E., Douglas, R. D., Hamilton, J. P. and Meyer, H. M. (1967). Rubella virus hemagglutination inhibition test. *New Engl. J. Med.* **276**, 554–557.

Straley, J. M. (1970) Disperse dyes. In *The Chemistry of Synthetic Dyes*, Vol. III (K. Venkataraman, ed), Academic Press, New York, pp. 385–462.

Strausser, H. (1959). Doctoral thesis, Rutgers University, New Brunswick, N.J.; *Dissert. Abstr.* **20**, 430.

Venkataraman, K. (ed.) (1977). *The Analytical Chemistry of Synthetic Dyes*, John Wiley, Chichester, p. 379.

Vyas, G. N. and Shulman, N. R. (1970), Hemagglutination assay for antigen and antibody associated with viral hepatitis. *Science* **170**, 332–333.

Wide, L. and Gemzell, C. A. (1960). An immunological pregnancy test. *Acta Endocr. Copenh.* **35**, 261–267.

CHAPTER 5

Immunoradiometric assays

T. S. Baker, S. R. Abbott, S. G. Daniel and J. F. Wright

Boots–Celltech Diagnostics Ltd,
240 Bath Road,
Slough, Berkshire SL1 4ET, UK

1. INTRODUCTION

The technique of radioimmunoassay (RIA), introduced by Yalow and Berson (1960), rapidly became established as a routine analytical method. Eight years later Miles and Hales (1968) proposed an alternative technique, the immunoradiometric assay (IRMA), citing its theoretical superiority over RIA. It is only in this decade, however, that these advantages have been demonstrated and IRMAs have begun to appear in routine clinical use.

1.1. The distinction between RIA and IRMA

In the conventional RIA [Fig. 1(a)], the substance to be estimated (analyte) competes with a radiolabelled analogue of the analyte (tracer) for a limited number of antibody binding sites. Thus the amount of tracer bound to antibody is inversely proportional to the concentration of analyte. By contrast, in the IRMA [Fig. 1(b)] the antibody is present in excess and carries the labelling isotope. Hence the amount of bound labelled antibody is in direct proportion to the amount of analyte. In the original form of the IRMA [Fig. 1(b)], as proposed by Miles and Hales, the remaining unreacted labelled antibody is removed by the addition of excess analyte coupled to solid phase

Analyte + Tracer* + Antibody → Analyte + Tracer* + Analyte + Tracer*
                                        | |
                                     Antibody   Antibody

(a)

Analyte + Antibody* → Analyte – Antibody* + Antibody*

(b)

Fig. 1. The principles of (a) RIA and (b) IRMA

(an immunoadsorbent, or ImAd). The supernatant containing the bound antibody can then be removed for counting.

In a subsequent development, Addison and Hales (1971) demonstrated a two-site IRMA in which the first antibody is coupled to a solid phase. This solid-phase reagent effectively 'extracts' the analyte from the solution. A second antibody, carrying the radioactive label and recognizing a second, distinct epitope on the antigen, is then added. Label is thus bound to the solid phase in direct proportion to the concentration of analyte (Fig. 2). The remaining 'free' label can be removed easily because the 'bound' complex is attached to a solid phase. The application of this two-site IRMA is obviously limited to analytes which are large enough simultaneously to bind two antibodies at different sites. Although this requirement precludes the measurement of haptens, there are still many analytes of clinical importance to which this assay principle may be applied advantageously.

Solid phase–Antibody$_1$ + Analyte → Solid phase–Antibody$_1$.Analyte

Solid phase–Antibody$_1$·Analyte + *Antibody$_2$ →

Solid phase–Antibody$_1$·Analyte·*Antibody$_2$ + *Antibody$_2$

Fig. 2. Two-site IRMA

In practice, the principle of the two-site IRMA has been modified to produce either an 'inclusive' assay, where both antibodies are added together, or a 'reverse' assay, where the analyte is reacted with the labelled antibody before the addition of the solid-phase antibody. In certain cases this delayed addition of antibody leads to an improvement in assay sensitivity.

1.2. Factors limiting the introduction of IRMAs

The main reason for the delay in IRMAs becoming more widely used is that the preparation of reagents, particularly labelled antibody, proved difficult prior to the availability of monoclonal antibodies. Unlike RIAs, IRMAs use excess antibody reagents and thus place considerable demands on the supply of pure materials. With polyclonal antisera as the sole source of antibody this demand can only be met by using immunopurification, which is difficult technically.

1.3. The impact of monoclonal antibodies

The rapid growth of monoclonal antibody technology (see Chapter 3 in this volume) has had a profound effect on the development of many immunoassays. The availability of monoclonal antibodies effectively removes the constraints of polyclonal antisera on the IRMA technique and provides an assured and essentially unlimited source of material for either radiolabelling (Section 2.1) or solid-phase preparation (Section 2.3). In practice, milligram quantities of purified monoclonal antibody are obtained from ascitic fluid or tissue culture and larger quantities of antibody for solid-phase preparation can be produced by scaling-up tissue culture systems (e.g. a 100 l air-lift fermenter is capable of yielding up to 5 g of purified monoclonal antibody in a single run).

2.   ADVANTAGES OF IRMA

The monoclonal antibody-based two-site IRMA offers significant advantages over RIA with respect to a number of important analytical features. These include the following:
(i) ease of radiolabelling; (ii) faster reaction rates; (iii) increased assay sensitivity; (iv) expanded working range; (v) higher specificity for analyte; (vi) improved assay robustness. These improvements will be discussed in turn.

2.1. Radiolabelling

Radiolabelling of antigens for RIA is often fraught with difficulties. Ideally, a pure homogeneous preparation of antigen is required, but there is often an inherent heterogeneity in biological substances, which may also be affected by conditions of purification and storage. Once a suitable preparation of antigen is available, it must be labelled without loss of immunoreactivity. However, iodination itself may produce additional heterogeneity, due to chemical or radiation damage. Furthermore, labelling the contaminants in an antigen preparation may adversely affect assay sensitivity. Radiolabelling of antigen is thus expensive in terms of both purified material and laboratory time.

One of the theoretical advantages of the IRMA is that it is the antibody, not the antigen, that is labelled. However, polyclonal antisera require affinity purification before they can be used to prepare a pure labelled reagent since hyperimmune animal sera generally yield less than 5% specific antibody in an immunoglobulin fraction.

With the advent of hybridization technology, large quantities of monoclonal antibodies of a consistent quality can now be produced. These reagents can be purified by standard procedures such as DEAE cellulose ion-exchange chromatography, protein A–Sepharose affinity chromatography and/or high performance liquid chromatography (HPLC). However, it should not be assumed that purity is assured by using a monoclonal antibody. Indeed, ascitic fluid usually contains significant amounts of non-specific mouse immunoglobulin and transferrin which readily co-purify, while hybridoma tissue culture supernatants may also contain variable amounts of ruminant immunoglobulin unless totally synthetic media are used. The presence of labelled contaminants in a labelled antibody reagent reduces the efficiency of IRMA. Quite apart from the spurious interference that labelled contaminants may exhibit in the antibody–antigen binding reaction, their additional contribution to non-specific binding (NSB) is highly detrimental. NSB tends to increase as the total mass of iodinated species increases. The use of high purity tracer ensures that the signal:noise ratio of the system is at a maximum.

Monoclonal antibodies usually iodinate efficiently without loss of immunoreactivity, for example using chloramine-T (Hunter and Greenwood, 1963), and the products are relatively stable. Assay sensitivity may be improved by increasing the specific activity of the labelled antibody, but this enhancement must be balanced against the rapid deterioration of immunoreactivity which is observed as the number of ^{125}I atoms introduced exceeds two per IgG molecule. The effect of radioiodination on immunoreactivity should always be checked (Hunter et al., 1983).

2.2. Reaction kinetics

The law of mass action predicts that the antibody–antigen binding reaction is driven to completion very rapidly when excess concentrations of antibody are present. Simpler kinetics also apply to a monoclonal antibody–single epitope reaction compared to a RIA or IRMA with polyclonal sera where a multiplicity of interactions are possible. Typically, IRMAs employing monoclonal antibodies in excess have reaction times of 2–3 h, whereas polyclonal antibody-based RIAs require 1–3 day incubation times to reach equilibrium. Thus IRMAs offer the convenience of within-day sample processing in the routine laboratory.

The use in an IRMA of excess reagents to drive the antibody–antigen reaction has certain other advantages. It is sometimes possible to obtain acceptable assay performance using relatively low affinity monoclonal antibodies, which perform only moderately well in corresponding RIA systems (Hunter *et al.*, 1984).

2.3. Assay sensitivity

A significant improvement in assay sensitivity (minimum detection limit) is one of the principal advantages of IRMA over RIA. The sensitivity of an assay system reflects the characteristics of the precision potential at low analyte concentration. Sensitivity may be defined as the concentration of analyte which corresponds to the mean plus 2.5 standard deviations of the response in the absence of analyte when interpolated from the dose–response curve.

In RIA, as demonstrated by Ekins (1981), sensitivity depends upon the experimental error and the inverse of the binding affinity of the antibody. In a two-site IRMA the detection limit depends upon the specific activity of the labelled antibody (Section 2.1), the affinity of the labelled antibody (and to a lesser extent the solid-phase antibody), and the degree of non-specific binding. It is the affinity of the labelled antibody that largely determines the position of the dose–response curve; the higher the affinity constant the more the curve shifts towards lower concentrations of analyte (Jackson *et al.*, 1983).

2.3.1. *'Signal to noise ratio'*

The concept of a 'signal to noise ratio' is useful when discussing assay performance with respect to sensitivity. Signal (analyte-dependent count rate) is a function of the specific activity of the labelled antibody reagent (Section 2.1) and the efficiency of the gamma-counter. Noise (analyte-independent count rate) depends on the counter background signal and the level of non-specific binding (NSB) of labelled antibody.

In a RIA only a fraction of the available analyte is involved in the response, since the amount of antibody is limited. By contrast, in an IRMA the use of excess antibody ensures that all the analyte takes part in signal generation. This advantage is particularly important at low levels of analyte and is partly responsible for the increased sensitivity that can be achieved by IRMA. As the amount of labelled antibody in the incubate increases so does sensitivity and, if NSB could be reduced to zero, optimal assay sensitivity would be achieved using an infinite amount of labelled antibody. In practice, however, increasing the amount of antibody also increases non-specific binding and an optimum must therefore be determined empirically so as to balance these two opposed effects.

In contrast to RIA systems, where high NSB levels compromise the top of the working range, high NSB values in an IRMA system decrease performance at the bottom of the range. Thus, lowering an IRMA's NSB has the effect of improving the signal to noise ratio of the system and hence the assay detection limit. This property allows the designer of the assay to obtain lower detection limits through judicious choice of an efficient separation stage.

2.3.2. The requirement for an efficient separation system

An important factor limiting the performance of all heterogeneous assay systems is the efficiency of the separation step. Assay precision and sensitivity both depend on a separation procedure which is precise, reproducible and gives minimal misclassification of the antibody-bound and free fractions. This aspect is particularly important with IRMAs because labelled antibody is present in excess so that any significant misclassification of the labelled material will increase NSB levels (and thus reduce assay sensitivity). Only with an extremely efficient separation system can the full analytical advantage of IRMAs be realized.

2.3.3. Solid-phase systems

The removal of unreacted labelled reagent is facilitated in the two-site IRMA by coupling one of the antibodies to a solid phase, so allowing the free label to be removed by washing. A wide variety of solid phases can be used. Some of the more common ones include plastic surfaces (coated tubes, microtitre plates, dipsticks or single polystyrene beads) to which antibodies adhere through non-covalent binding. However, these solid phases tend to suffer from both limited capacity and inconsistency due to batch variations, and may also be subject to loss of coating antibody if the non-covalent bonds are unstable. Small, finely dispersed particles such as microcrystalline cellulose, glass or polymeric monodisperse particles may also be used as solid phases. These have the advantage of higher binding capacity and, where covalent coupling is employed, more stable linkage with the antibody.

Between these two extremes lie the medium size particles, e.g. Sephadex, Sepharose and Sephacryl. These materials are porous and have a high capacity for the covalent coupling of antibody, but settle relatively quickly and require agitation during incubation.

2.3.4. Separation systems

The method of separation of the free and solid phase-bound fractions obviously varies with the nature of the materials. With coated tubes, beads or microtitre wells, simple repeated washing can be employed, but this procedure may be labour-intensive if large numbers of samples are involved. With finely divided particles which stay in suspension, repeated centrifugation and suspension in a wash solution is required—again a fairly laborious affair unless expensive modifications are made to centrifuges and aspirating–washing equipment. More recent developments in this area include the use of magnetic particles which sediment when a magnetic field generated by rare earth magnets is applied, but again extensive washing of the solid phase is required.

The sucrose layering method is a separation system which overcomes many of these difficulties (Wright and Hunter, 1983). For this method (Fig. 3), the solid phase must be of medium size and density (e.g. Sephacryl) such that it will settle relatively quickly under gravity, removing the need for centrifugation. The technique involves the controlled layering of a relatively dense sucrose solution below the pre-diluted assay incubate. This procedure raises the incubate, including the solid-phase material, within the reaction tube. After 15 min the solid phase-bound fraction settles through the sucrose leaving the incubate with remaining free labelled material in the upper layer. This passage of the solid-phase material through the sucrose results in efficient washing. The upper layer of incubate and most of the sucrose are aspirated to waste, leaving all the solid phase in the bottom of the tube. After a repeat of this process, NSB in a two-site IRMA can be reduced to as little as 0.1–0.2% of the total label added. As there is no loss of the solid phase, very sensitive assays with high precision may be obtained. The technique is convenient to perform and may be applied to a large number of samples.

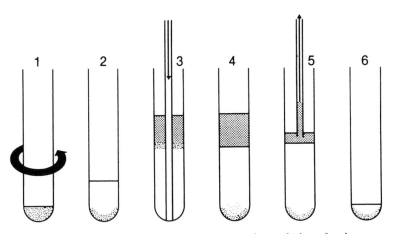

Fig. 3. The principle of the SUCROSEP* sucrose layering technique for the separation of free and bound fractions in solid-phase immunoassays. Steps: 1, solid phase is agitated during incubation; 2, wash buffer is added; 3, relatively dense sucrose solution is introduced; 4, solid phase is allowed to settle, 5, upper layer (free fraction) is removed to waste; 6, solid phase (bound fraction) is counted for radioactivity

*SUCROSEP is a trademark of Boots-Celltech Diagnostics Ltd.

2.3.5. Clinical significance of improved IRMA sensitivity

Assay sensitivity is a factor limiting the application of many immunoassays in clinical chemistry. A prime example is the immunoassay of human thyrotropin (TSH). Normal circulating levels of TSH are low and conventional RIAs for the hormone are unable to detect the full range of values. The use of basal TSH determinations by RIAs is therefore limited to the distinction of elevated values from normal. Monoclonal antibody-based TSH IRMAs with efficient separation systems have sensitivities increased by an order of magnitude relative to existing RIAs. A typical dose–response curve for the SUCROSEP TSH IRMA, which has a sensitivity of 0.06 mIU l^{-1}TSH, is shown in Fig. 4. The introduction of sensitive TSH IRMAs offers to extend the use of basal measurements of the hormone concentration to the differentiation of hyperthyroidism from euthyroidism.

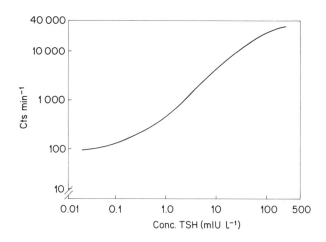

Fig. 4. A typical dose–response curve for the SUCROSEP TSH IRMA

2.4. Working range

The working range of an immunoassay can be defined arbitrarily as the range of analyte concentrations with an intra-assay coefficient of variation (CV) of less than 10%. RIAs typically have narrow working ranges covering only two to three orders of analyte concentration. Since the pathophysiological range of many serum analytes occurs over three or more orders of concentration, it is often necessary to run samples in RIAs at more than one dilution. IRMAs, by contrast, often have working ranges covering three to four orders of concentration so that sample dilution is unnecessary.

2.4.1. Precision profile

An effective way to describe both intra- and inter-assay precision is as a profile (precision potential) which relates the CV of the response to analyte concentration, and is characteristically a U-shaped plot (Ekins, 1976). The precision profile for an IRMA is typically both broader (wider working range) and reaches a lower nadir (increased precision) than the corresponding RIA. This improved working range of IRMAs relative to RIA is illustrated by the precision profiles shown in Fig. 5.

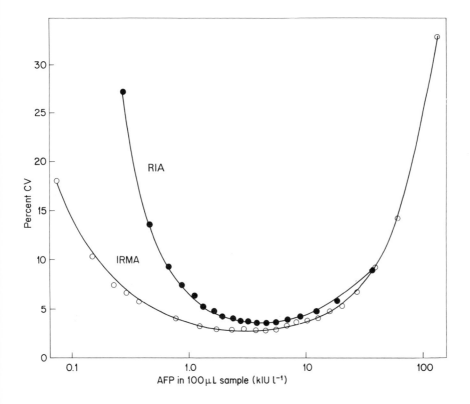

Fig. 5. A comparison of precision profiles for an AFP RIA and an AFP IRMA using the same antiserum and separation system (sucrose layering system). Total incubation times were 3 h for the IRMA and 20 h for the RIA. [From W.M. Hunter and P.C. Budd, *Journal of Immunological Methods*, **45**, 225–273 (1981), reproduced by permission of Elsevier/North Holland Biomedical Press]

2.4.2. 'High-dose Hook' effect

A feature which potentially limits the working range of IRMAs is the so-called 'high-dose hook' effect. This is the tendency in an inclusive or reverse two-site IRMA for the dose–response curve to invert at extremely high doses of analyte, an effect not seen in RIA. The hook effect occurs because solid phase-bound antibody becomes limiting at high analyte concentrations, so that free analyte begins to compete with the analyte-labelled antibody complex for solid phase. The 'hook region' can effectively be set at higher analyte concentrations by increasing the concentration of solid phase-bound antibody, and in well optimized IRMAs it occurs at values well outside the pathophysiological range. Any potential confusion caused by extremely high levels of analyte can be avoided by assaying the sample at more than one dilution.

2.5. Specificity

The specificity of RIA is a simple function of the ability of other substances to cross-react with the antibody. Cross-reactants compete with labelled antigen for binding to antibody and thus always act to reduce binding giving rise to a positive bias in measurement of analyte. Cross-reactivity is normally quantified as the amount of cross-reacting compound required to produce a given displacement of tracer, relative to the amount of analyte required to give the same displacement.

As two antibodies are involved in a two-site IRMA, each with its own characteristics, the specificity of an assay reflects two separate phenomena, cross-reactivity and interference. Furthermore, since the antibodies are in excess, the effects of any non-specificity may be accentuated in an IRMA.

2.5.1. Interference

In a two-site IRMA, a substance may bind to one antibody of the pair, but not to the other. If so, the amount of labelled antibody bound for a given analyte concentration decreases as the concentration of interfering substance increases. This interference results in *negative* bias in the measurement of analyte.

An IRMA system can be tested for interference by studying the recovery of analyte in the presence of high concentrations of the potential interfering substance. Possible interference by the glycoprotein hormones LH, FSH and hCG was studied in the SUCROSEP TSH IRMA in this manner (Table 1). It may be seen that there was no significant interference of TSH measurement by LH or FSH in the IRMA. However, hCG did cause limited interference resulting in an ~13% decrease in the concentration of TSH detected. This

Table 1. Interference in SUCROSEP TSH IRMA

Hormone	Hormone concentration (IU l^{-1})	Expected TSH (mIU l^{-1})	Observed TSH (mIU l^{-1})	Interference $\left(\dfrac{\text{observed TSH conc.}}{\text{expected TSH conc.}}\right)$
LH	60	3.93	3.94	1.00
FSH	32	3.93	3.84	0.98
hCG	50 000	3.93	3.41	0.87

effect can be explained by competition between hCG and TSH for binding to one of the antibodies in the system such that some of the analyte binding capacity is lost.

2.5.2. Cross-reactivity

When a substance is capable of binding simultaneously to both the labelled antibody and the solid phase-bound antibody in an IRMA system, then bridging of the two antibodies is possible in the absence of analyte. This phenomenon, referred to here as cross-reactivity, results in an increase in binding and *positive* bias in the measurement of analyte.

Cross-reactivity in an IRMA may be assessed by measuring the response to increasing doses of potential cross-reactant at zero analyte concentration, and was studied in the SUCROSEP TSH IRMA (Table 2). There appeared to be some cross-reactivity with prolactin, LH and FSH, but these effects were probably due to contamination of the reference preparations with TSH. This explanation is supported by two observations: (i) that hCG, from a urinary

Table 2. Cross-reactivity in SUCROSEP TSH IRMA

Hormone	Hormone concentration (IU l^{-1})	Expected TSH (mIU l^{-1})	Observed TSH (mIU l^{-1})	Cross-reactivity $\left(\dfrac{\text{apparent mass TSH}}{\text{mass cross-reactant}}\right)$
Bovine TSH	100	0	Undetectable	None
Growth Hormone	0.32	0	Undetectable	None
Prolactin	3.2	0	1.06	0.004
LH	60	0	0.13	0.009
FSH	32	0	0.06	0.004
hCG	50 000	0	Undetectable	None

extract, did not cross-react though it is structurally very similar to TSH, LH and FSH, and (ii) that there was no cross-reactivity with growth hormone of recombinant DNA origin, even though it is structurally related to prolactin.

2.5.3. Monoclonal antibody selection and epitope analysis

During the development of a two-site IRMA, monoclonal antibodies are often selected initially on the basis of their specificity in RIA. Once a panel of suitable antibodies has been selected, epitope analysis may be carried out. This procedure effectively determines which pairs of monoclonals can be used successfully together as labelled antibody and solid phase reagent. Pairs of monoclonal antibodies which together show good dose–response characteristics must recognize different epitopes which are spatially separated on the analyte molecule.

2.5.4. Assays for molecular conformation and structure

The exquisite specificity potential of monoclonal antibodies allows the molecular structure of an antigen to be probed in detail, and the appropriate selection of antibodies for IRMA, whether fortuitous or judicious, sometimes leads to interesting observations. Two examples serve to illustrate this point. In an IRMA for human luteinizing hormone (LH) the epitope recognized by a selected antibody was shown to share structures on both the α and β subunits, since the IRMA reacted to the intact hormone, but not to either of the individual subunits (Hunter et al., 1984). If this antibody is used, the LH IRMA is specific for intact LH, i.e. for the natural conformation of the intact hormone. A second example concerns a two-site IRMA for interferon-α (IFN-α) developed using a solid-phase polyclonal anti-IFN-α antiserum and one of a pair of monoclonal antibodies to IFN-α (NK2 or YOK 5/19). In man, IFN-α comprises a family of structurally related subtypes, each the product of a separate gene. The subtype recognition characteristics of the IRMA using either ^{125}I-NK2 or ^{125}I-YOK 5/19 are shown in Fig. 6, and it may be seen that the substitution of one labelled monoclonal antibody for the other reverses the relative potency of the IRMA for IFN-α_1 and IFN-α_2. The careful selection of a panel of anti-IFN-α monoclonal antibodies with appropriate restricted subtype recognition profiles should thus allow the IFN-α subtype composition of a natural IFN-α preparation to be analysed, a task beyond the capability of either biological assays or radioimmunoassays for IFN.

2.5.5. Problems of 'over-specificity'

In certain situations, it may be envisaged that a conventional two-site IRMA will exhibit too narrow a specificity. In such situations it may be necessary to

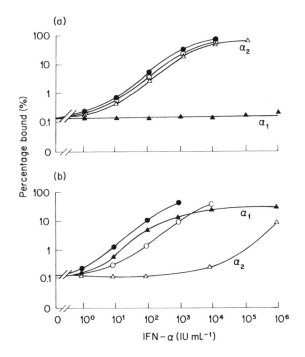

Fig. 6. Interferon (IFN) sub-type recognition characteristics of an IFN-α IRMA using (a) ^{125}I-NK2 monoclonal antibody and (b) ^{125}I-YOK 5/19 monoclonal antibody. Circles denote natural IFN-α preparations, triangles denote IFN-α of recombinant DNA origin.

mix monoclonal antibodies so as to effect a broader assay specificity. If such an approach is adopted, close attention must be given to differences in kinetics which may apply to the component monoclonal antibodies.

The calibration of specific monoclonal antibody-based IRMAs may be difficult if the reference standard contains a variety of molecular species or fragments. However, if the monoclonal antibodies selected detect only the biologically active components of the standard, this should be a distinct advantage and will result in improved correlation between the biological activity and immunoreactivity of reference preparations. Indeed, with the application of highly specific monoclonal antibody-based IRMAs, the validity of certain reference preparations may well be thrown into question.

2.5.6. Limitations to the application of the two-site IRMA

It is generally thought that an epitope corresponds to five or six amino acids and so the minimum theoretical size of an analyte which can be measured in a two-site IRMA is probably 10–12 amino acids. However, allowing for conformation and possible steric hindrance between two antibodies binding simultaneously to such a small polypeptide, the minimum size is probably somewhat greater.

2.6. Robustness

In the context of immunoassay, robustness is an all embracing term used to describe the stability of an assay system to variations in the protocol and local environment. These changes can occur, for instance, when an assay is performed by different laboratories or different operators. It is generally accepted that the increased robustness of IRMAs is one of their most significant advantages. We will discuss this feature with respect to a number of possible variables.

2.6.1. Temperature

RIA relies on the attainment of an equilibrium which is itself dependent upon the affinity constant of the antibody. As such, RIAs are subject to severe thermodynamic constraints and are very susceptible to temperature changes. However, in IRMA, the large excess of antibody essentially drives the reaction towards completion, so that the assay is far less susceptible to temperature variations. A well designed IRMA can often be performed at temperatures as disparate as 4 °C and 37 °C without significant effect.

2.6.2. pH and ionic strength

In practice monoclonal antibodies exhibit rather narrow pH and ionic strength activity profiles compared to polyclonal antibodies. Therefore these characteristics have to be thoroughly studied during the development of a two-site IRMA. In a two-site IRMA, appropriate buffers must be employed which are compatible with both monoclonal antibodies if assay robustness is to be assured.

2.6.3. Matrix effects

Samples of serum or plasma constitute complex biological mixtures, but may conveniently be considered as consisting of the analyte and the matrix. Certain components of the matrix can interfere non-specifically with the immune binding reaction of an immunoassay. The factors responsible for this effect are still largely unknown, but almost certainly include circulating proteins and lipids. In general, matrix effects seem to be less pronounced in monoclonal antibody-based IRMAs than in RIAs, probably because the former require simple bimolecular reactions rather than the complex lattice formation associated with polyclonal antisera.

To compensate for matrix effects, standard solutions of the analyte are generally made up in an analyte-free biological fluid pool, equivalent to the fluid on which the assay is to be performed. For example, if the assay is to be performed on human serum then analyte free human serum may be used. A convenient alternative approach is to employ a diluent based on non-primate animal serum. A suitable formulation may be determined empirically so that the dose–response achieved in such a diluent is superimposable on that for human serum.

An exacting test of an assay's robustness with respect to variations in sample, is to determine the recovery of exogenous analyte added to a series of samples. In such a test, a mean recovery of ~100% indicates that the matrices of the samples and standards are equivalent. If, in addition, the exogenous analyte is a reference preparation and is added quantitatively to the test sera, such an investigation also provides a measure of the assay's accuracy. Recovery data typical of a well optimized two-site IRMA are shown in Table 3.

Table 3. Recovery of exogenous TSH from individual sera

TSH added (mIU l^{-1})	No. of samples	Mean recovery (%)	S.D.	CV (%)
0.54	20	100.5	15.4	15.3
5.82	20	99.4	3.1	3.1
12.2	20	95.5	3.8	4.0
24.4	20	95.6	3.4	3.6
57.1	20	104.8	5.3	5.1

In a two-site IRMA system, especially one employing monoclonal antibodies, positive bias can arise due to the presence of circulating anti-immunoglobulin antibodies in the sera of certain individuals. These may cross-react with mouse antibody and, because of their bifunctional nature, form bridging complexes between solid phase-bound antibody and labelled antibody. This artefact can easily be abolished by inclusion of an appropriate animal serum in the system.

2.6.4. Pipetting precision

RIAs normally have at least three critical pipetting stages (sample, antibody and tracer) and imprecise addition of any of these solutions increases the variability of the assay. In contrast, because both labelled and solid phase-bound antibody reagents are in excess, IRMAs generally have only one critical volume-dependent stage—sample pipetting.

3. THE FUTURE OF IRMA IN CLINICAL CHEMISTRY

3.1. Assay data handling

With the emergence of immunoassays as important routine methods in clinical chemistry, and the availability of computing facilities, there has been increasing interest in the development of computer programs to process immunoassay data. Statistical approaches to curve fitting and data analysis have also been widely discussed (e.g. IAEA, 1982; Hunter and Corrie, 1983). The greater analytical potential of IRMA will demand a greater sophistication in both statistical analysis and curve fitting. However, this movement must be tempered by the need for general application to available microcomputers.

To make the best use of IRMA data, a balance must be achieved between flexibility of the curve fitting algorithm and the selection and rejection of outlying data (Malan, 1982). Thus, spline curve fitting methods are too flexible, while linear logit–log transforms are generally too rigid. An acceptable compromise, albeit more complex, is offered by the four-parameter log–logistic model (Healy, 1972). This method is restricted, however, to use with a dose–response curve which is symmetrical about the point of inflection. With improved separation, IRMA response curves are in fact asymmetric. Processing of IRMA data with a four-parameter logistic model can, therefore, lead to variable bias of results across the dose range.

This problem can be overcome by using a five-parameter logistic model (Rodbard et al., 1978)–the fifth parameter being a measure of the degree of asymmetry of the response curve. This type of model has been incorporated into the well received Edinburgh Immunoassay Package (Raab and McKenzie, 1981; McKenzie and Thompson, 1983).

At present the most widely used automated data processing programs are those supplied with counting equipment, and these have generally been restricted to use with RIA data. Data reduction programs both capable of processing IRMA data and compatible with microcomputers are now becoming available. This trend will certainly continue.

3.2. Automation

As in other areas of clinical chemistry, there is a growing movement towards automation of immunoassays. Solid-phase IRMAs appear to be inherently better suited to eventual automation than do RIAs. Their rapid kinetics allow the use of non-equilibrium reactions without the penalty of significant assay drift. This advantage, together with the application of non-centrifugation separation techniques, promises to allow the development of automated systems capable of high sample throughput without the use of over-elaborate instrumentation.

3.3. Sensitivity

The theoretical detection limit of IRMAs are, in part, set by the the affinity constant of the selected antibodies. To date, the monoclonal antibodies used in two-site IRMAs typically have affinity constants of 10^9-10^{11} l mol^{-1}, so that judicious selection of antibodies with higher affinities (up to 10^{12} l mol $^{-1}$) is likely to improve assay sensitivity still further. However, with well selected antibodies, assay sensitivity is ultimately limited by the constraints of signal generation, i.e. by the specific activity of the radiolabel, and in situations where this limit becomes significant, further progress must ultimately lie with non-isotopic immunoassays.

3.4. A challenge to non-isotopic immunometric assays

This chapter has attempted to highlight the benefits of the two-site IRMA as an alternative to RIA. Although most clinical chemistry laboratories routinely carry out RIA and, therefore, have the necessary γ-counters available for IRMA, immunometric assays employing alternative end-points clearly have certain advantages, and these are the subject of other chapters in this volume.

The increasing deployment of two-site IRMAs has set a high standard for immunoassay performance. These merits will have to be at least equalled by non-isotopic assay systems before the latter become routinely adopted in the clinical chemistry laboratory. It seems likely that two-site IRMAs will remain a realistic alternative immunoassay system for the clinical chemistry laboratory for a number of years to come and will provide a high standard of performance by which novel assay methods may be assessed.

ACKNOWLEDGEMENTS

We wish to acknowledge our debt to our former colleague, Dr W. M. Hunter, whose work underlies much that is described here. We are also grateful to Angela Symes for her expert assistance in preparing this contribution.

NOTE ADDED IN PROOF

It has now been shown that prolactin of non-pituitary origin does not cross-react in the SUCROSEP TSH IRMA.

REFERENCES

Addison, G. M. and Hales, C. N. (1971). In *Radioimmunoassay Methods* K. E. Kirkham and W. M. Hunter, eds), Churchill Livingstone, Edinburgh, pp. 481–487.

Ekins, R. P. (1976). General principles of hormone assay. In *Hormone Assays and Their Clinical Application* (J. A. Loraine and E. T. Bell, eds), Churchill Livingstone, Edinburgh, pp. 1–72.

Ekins, R. P. (1981). Towards immunoassays of greater sensitivity, specificity and speed: an overview. In *Monoclonal Antibodies and Development in Immunoassay* (A. Albertini and R. P. Ekins, eds), pp. 1–21.

Healy, M. J. R. (1972). Statistical analysis of radioimmunoassay data. *Biochem. J.* **130**, 207–210.

Hunter, W. M. and Greenwood, F. C. (1963). Preparation of iodine-131 labelled human growth hormone of high specific activity. *Nature, Lond.* **194**, 495–496.

Hunter, W. M. and Corrie, J. E. T. (eds) (1983). *Immunoassays for Clinical Chemistry*, Churchill Livingstone, Edinburgh, pp. 597–665.

Hunter, W. M., Bennie, J. G., Budd, P. S., van Heyningen, V., James, K., Micklem, R. I. and Scott, A. (1983). Immunoradiometric assays using monoclonal antibodies. In *Immunoassays for Clinical Chemistry* (W. M. Hunter and J. E. T. Corrie, eds), Churchill Livingstone, Edinburgh, pp. 531–544.

Hunter, W. M., Bennie, J. G., Kellett, H. A., Micklem, L. R., Scott, A. and James, K. (1984). A monoclonal antibody-based immunoradiometric assay for h-LH. *Ann. Clin. Biochem.* **21**, 275–283.

IAEA (1983). *Radioimmunoassay and Related Procedures in Medicine*, IAEA, Vienna, pp. 383–444.

Jackson, T. M., Marshall, N. J. and Ekins, R. P. (1983). Optimisation of immunoradiometric (labelled antibody) assays. In *Immunoassays for Clinical Chemistry* (W. M. Hunter and J. E. T. Corrie, eds). Churchill Livingstone, Edinburgh, pp. 557–575.

Malan, P. G. (1982). Immunoassay data-processing and quality control error analysis. *RIA Design* (J. I. Thorell, ed.), Pegasus Press, Paris, pp. 45–58.

McKenzie, I. G. M. and Thompson, R. C. H. (1983). Design and implementation of a software package for analysis of immunoassay data. In *Immunoassays for Clinical Chemistry* (W. M. Hunter and J. E. T. Corrie, eds), Churchill Livingstone, Edinburgh, pp. 608–613.

Miles, L. E. M. and Hales, C. N. (1968). Labelled antibodies and immunological assay systems. *Nature, Lond.* **219**, 186–189.

Raab, G. I. and McKenzie, I. G. M. (1981). A modular program for processing immunoassay data. In *Quality Control in Clinical Endocrinology: Proceedings of the 8th Tenovus Workshop* (D. W. Wilson, S. J. Gaskell, and K. Kemp, eds), Alpha Omega Press, Cardiff, pp. 225–236.

Rodbard, D., Munsen, P. J. and DeLean, A. (1978). Improved curve-fitting, parallelism testing, characterization of sensitivity and specificity, validation and optimization for radiological assays. In *Radioimmunoassay and Related Procedures in Medicine*, Vol. 1, IAEA, Vienna, pp. 469–503.

Wright, J. F. and Hunter, W. M. (1983). The sucrose layering separation: a non-centrifugation system. In *Immunoassays for Clinical Chemistry* (W. M. Hunter and J. E. T. Corrie, eds). Churchill Livingstone, Edinburgh, pp. 170–177.

Yallow, R. S. and Benson, S. A. (1960) Immunoassay of endogenous plasma insulin in man. *J. Clin. Invest.* **39**, 1157–1175.

Alternative Immunoassays
Edited by W. P. Collins
© 1985 John Wiley & Sons Ltd

CHAPTER 6

Enzyme immunoassays

A. Voller†‡ and D. E. Bidwell†

† *Immunodiagnostics Unit,*
  Nuffield Laboratories of Comparative Medicine,
  Institute of Zoology,
  The Zoological Society of London,
  Regents Park, London NW1 4RY, UK
  and
‡ *Department of Clinical Tropical Medicine,*
  London School of Hygiene and Tropical Medicine,
  Keppel Street, London WC1E 7HT, UK

1. INTRODUCTION

For the purposes of this article we will consider enzyme immunoassays as those methods in which enzymes are used to determine antibodies, antigens or haptens. In practice this usually means that an enzyme-labelled immunoreagent (equivalent to the isotopic label in radioimmunoassay) is used and that its presence and level can be monitored by means of coloured, fluorescent, or chemiluminescent substrates or by changes in pH or conductivity. Other people may classify immunoassays on the basis of the signal detected, e.g. fluorescence, chemiluminescence, etc., so there will be a certain degree of overlapping. The nomenclature is extremely confusing at present and is worsening year by year.

Enzyme immunoassays can be further subdivided into two major groups:

(i) *Homogeneous (non-separation) assays* In these methods the enzyme activity is altered by the immunological reaction when the carrier of the enzyme participates in an antigen–antibody reaction (e.g. EMIT, Syva Corp., USA).

(ii) *Heterogeneous (separation) assays* In these assays the enzyme activity is unaltered by antigen–antibody reactions. Thus in the heterogeneous systems reacted antibody or antigen must be separated from the unreacted components whereas in the homogeneous assays no such separation is needed.

2. HOMOGENEOUS ENZYME IMMUNOASSAYS

One of the earliest of these assays was the enzyme-multiplied immunoassay test (EMIT) (Curtiss and Patel, 1978; Oellerich, 1980). In this method small molecules (usually drugs) are labelled with an enzyme. When specific antibody is reacted with the enzyme–hapten conjugate the enzymatic activity is altered; in fact it is usually reduced. The effect of the antibody will be reversed by free hapten in the test samples. Thus in this method reference antibody and reference hapten–enzyme conjugate are mixed with the test sample and the results compared with those obtained when the same reagents are mixed with hapten-free samples and with known amounts of haptens. The more drug that is present in the test sample the more enzymatic activity is retained and so the more coloured product is generated.

These assays will not be considered in detail, but they have been commercialized by the Syva Corporation for many drugs of abuse, cardiovascular drugs and anti-epileptics. The EMIT assays are usually restricted to the measurement of small molecules and the sensitivity is usually in the microgram per millilitre range. However, more recently an EMIT-type assay for IgG has been reported and the sensitivity is adequate (Gibbons *et al.*, 1980).

2.1. Substrate-labelled fluorescent immunoassay (SLFIA)

In this method a fluorescent enzyme substrate is bound to an antigen or hapten. The complex is not fluorescent, but after hydrolysis with an appropriate enzyme the product will fluoresce. The fluorescence will not occur in the presence of antibody to the hapten. The test is carried out by mixing the sample (which may contain the drug hapten) with the substrate-labelled hapten and the reference antibody with enzyme. Increasing amounts of hapten in the sample lead to high fluorescence values.

Again this method is rather insensitive, but it is rapid and simple (Wong *et al.*, 1979) and has been adapted for protein estimations (Ngo *et al.*, 1981). Reagents for the measurement of theophylline have been attached to a paper matrix on a dipstick (Greenquist *et al.*, 1981).

2.2. Apoenzyme reactivation immunoassay (ARIS)

The flavin N^6-(N^1-2,4-dinitrophenol-6-aminohexyl) adenine dinucleotide (DNP-FAD) has been used as a label in competitive binding assays for various drugs. The labelled ligand not bound to antibody acts as a prosthetic group for glucose oxidase apoenzyme, which reacts with glucose and oxygen through a peroxidase-linked system to generate a colour, which is proportional to the hapten concentration. The method for the measurement of theophylline has been adapted to a reagent-strip format (Tyhach et al., 1981).

2.3. Enzyme channelling immunoassay

In this approach beads are coated with two different enzymes. The product of one of the enzymes is the substrate for the other. In this assay for antigen, agarose coated with one enzyme and the antigen is incubated with the test sample containing analyte and a second enzyme-labelled antibody. Sensitivity was in the nanogram per millilitre range for IgG (Litman et al., 1980). Subsequently, the reagents for the measurement of morphine have been attached to a test strip and a sensitivity of ~ 30 pg ml^{-1} has been achieved (Litman et al., 1983).

3. HETEROGENEOUS ENZYME IMMUNOASSAYS

In these assays, enzyme-labelled antibody conjugates are usually employed (although labelled antigen can be used) and the essential point to note is that the enzyme activity is not altered during the immunological reaction. In fact the main objective is to preserve as much activity as possible in both the enzyme and antibody in the conjugate. The best known of these assays is the enzyme-linked immunosorbent assay (ELISA) which combines the virtues of solid-phase technology with the merits of an enzyme-labelled immuno-reagent (Engvall and Perlmann, 1971).

Virtually all radioimmunoassays (RIAs) are based on the concept of competition for specific antibody between a limited amount of a labelled reference antigen or hapten with the analyte in the test sample. Some of the earliest ELISA methods were also of this limited reagent type, probably because the users at that time were endocrinologists who were accustomed to the conventional RIA approaches (Van Weeman and Schuurs, 1972). Since that time there has been a decisive and progressive movement towards ELISA tests based on excess labelled reagent (usually labelled antibody) methods. Typically these assays are multilayer sandwich or immunometric methods; for example, the most usual formats for antigen assays are as indicated in Fig. 1.

This sandwich approach is particularly useful for assaying antigens in complex mixtures, since the wash step after each incubation removes all heterologous materials which might interfere with the assay. This immunometric approach has been found to have the same accuracy as conventional competitive methods and means that the assays can be used even when high precision is required. The method is also suitable for those tests where a yes/no answer is all that is required, and in such instances the results can be

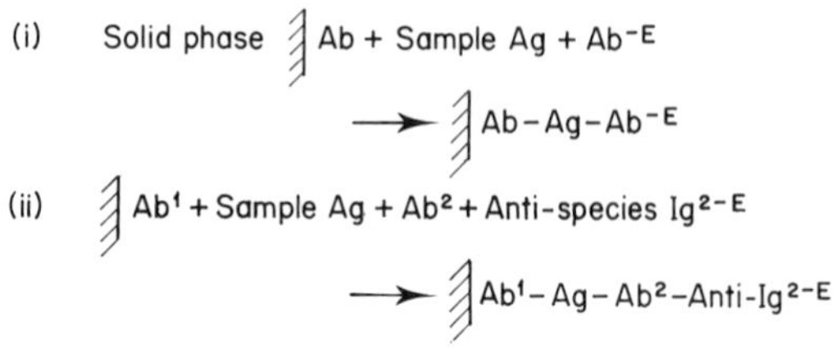

(i)   Solid phase ζ Ab + Sample Ag + Ab^{-E}

$\longrightarrow$ ζ Ab – Ag – Ab^{-E}

(ii) ζ Ab^1 + Sample Ag + Ab^2 + Anti-species Ig^{2-E}

$\longrightarrow$ ζ Ab^1 – Ag – Ab^2 – Anti-Ig^{2-E}

Fig. 1. The principles of immunometric assays, E, enzyme

read visually. ELISA tests for hepatitis B surface antigen and other hepatitis markers have proved particularly successful, as have those tests for rotavirus which can be carried out directly on faecal samples without pretreatment (for reviews see Voller et al., 1979; Voller and Bidwell, 1980).

These methods have had most widespread use in detecting infectious diseases where RIA never became firmly established. Currently the ELISA is also replacing the reverse passive agglutination tests, which were widely used for infectious disease antigens. The fact that objective results can be obtained in a test with stable reagents and in formats permitting batch processing (of 50–100 samples per unit) means that the ELISA is very suitable for screening (e.g. as in blood banks or for epidemiological purposes).

These immunometric assays require that the antigen has at least two reactive antigenic sites. These can have the same specificity, in which case the same antibody can be used for both coating the solid phase and for the conjugate. However, most infectious agents have multiple antigenic sites of different specificities and it is now possible to produce monoclonal antibodies to those different antigens. This permits the ELISA to be reformulated as shown in Fig. 2.

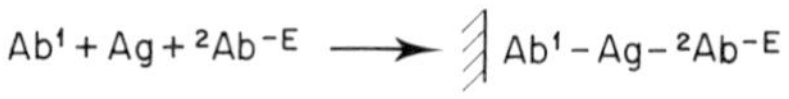

Ab^1 + Ag + ^{2}Ab^{-E} $\longrightarrow$ ζ Ab^1 – Ag – ^{2}Ab^{-E}

Fig. 2. A modified immunometric assay

This approach means that both the sample and labelled antibody can be added together to the solid phase, thus eliminating one incubation step. These 'one-step' assays can give high specificity by virtue of the two different antigenic sites involved and they can be quick and convenient. It is probable that in the future many of the assays for infectious diseases will be of this type.

The procedure may also be carried out in two steps (see Chapter 5 in this volume) and sensitive immunoenzymometric assays have been developed for

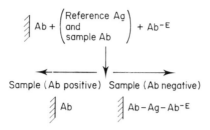

Fig. 3. Inhibition, immunometric assay

the measurement of hCG, hLH and hTSH using alkaline phosphatase as the label (Wada *et al.*, 1982). More recently the methods for hCG and hLH have been presented as dipsticks.

It is also possible to measure antibody by inhibiting the detection of antigen in any of the above-mentioned assays (Fig. 3).

The degree of inhibition of antigen uptake by the solid phase is proportional to the amount of antibody in the test sample. This approach can be useful when it is impossible or difficult to prepare a purified antigen. However, if such an antigen can be made then the indirect method using labelled antiglobulin is preferable (Fig. 4).

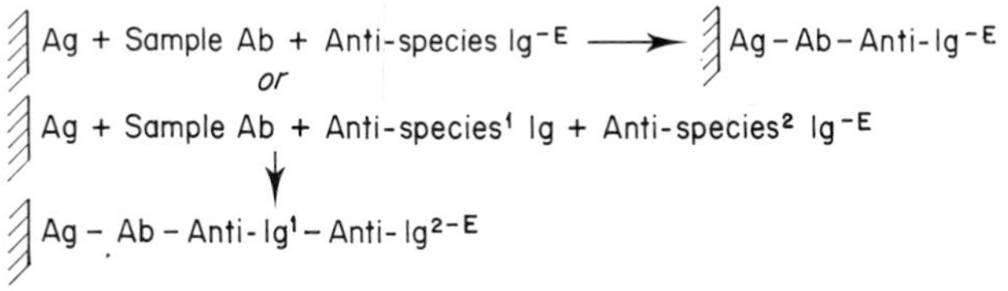

Ag + Sample Ab + Anti-species Ig^{-E} $\longrightarrow$ Ag – Ab – Anti-Ig^{-E}
or
Ag + Sample Ab + Anti-species^1 Ig + Anti-species^2 Ig^{-E}

Ag – Ab – Anti-Ig^1 – Anti-Ig^{2-E}

Fig. 4. Some immunometric assays using solid phase-bound antigen

In this modification only a single conjugate, e.g. enzyme-labelled anti-rabbit IgG, will be needed to measure antibodies in a wide variety of species against whose immunoglobulin rabbit antisera have been made. It is also possible to use enzyme-labelled protein A instead of anti-species immunoglobulin.

This sandwich or indirect method for antibody detection and measurement has been used extensively, especially in microbiology. Indirect ELISA tests are available for the measurement of antibodies to virtually all viruses, bacteria, parasites of human and veterinary importance and has to a large degree replaced complement fixation, haemagglutination and microscopical immunofluorescence. Most of the tests are in the microplate format which permits easy testing of large numbers of samples, but which is less convenient for individual tests where single or strips of microwells, beads or pegs have the advantage.

There is growing interest in the detection of immunoglobulin class-specific antibody, especially of the IgM class. The indirect method as shown above can sometimes be effective, but false positives can occur in the presence of IgG antibody and IgM anti-IgG rheumatoid factor and false negatives can occur due to competition of IgM with high levels of IgG antibody. The antibody class capture assay approach can overcome these problems (Fig. 5).

This format permits an immuno-separation of the serum during the test procedure and the specificity is imparted by the antigen and labelled specific antibody. The approach has been most successful for the detection of hepatitis A IgM.

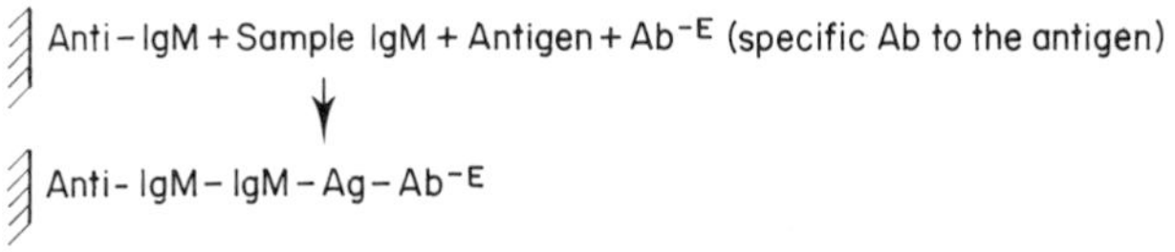

Anti – IgM + Sample IgM + Antigen + Ab^{-E} (specific Ab to the antigen)

↓

Anti- IgM – IgM – Ag – Ab^{-E}

Fig. 5. An antibody class capture immunoassay

Although ELISA has been used predominantly for large analytes and all the above approaches are dependent upon multi-antigenic sites, it is also possible to measure haptens by inhibition ELISA methods (Fig. 6).

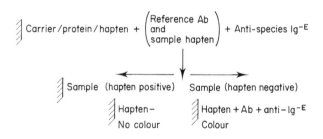

Fig. 6. An ELISA for the measurement of haptens

This method is dependent upon the antibody being made with a second carrier protein, different to that used to link the hapten to the solid phase. Various modifications can be made (e.g. to label the antibody with enzyme rather than use labelled antiglobulin). One advantage of this approach is that labelled antibody is used. There is now a vast body of literature on enzyme labelling of antibodies and a single procedure can be used in contrast to the many types of methods needed to label individual haptens. This inhibition method has been used for the measurement of drugs and the sensitivity is at least as high as that obtained with conventional RIA (Niewola et al., 1983). More recently an enzyme-labelled immunometric assay has been reported for the measurement of digoxin (Freytag et al., 1984).

4. COMPONENTS OF ELISA SYSTEMS

Up to this point we have dealt with ELISA in the generic sense without regard to the variety of label and detection methods that can be used. If we are dealing with RIA there are few labels (essentially ^{125}I and ^{3}H), so the choice is limited, as is the detection method. However, in ELISA we can use virtually any enzyme that can be linked to an immuno-reagent. Clearly it has to be stable, have a high turnover rate and be cheap, with a suitable substrate. Even so, the range goes from alkaline phosphatase, β-galactosidase, peroxidase, glucose oxidase to urease and penicillinase, to name but a few. The choice has to be made with the detection method in mind. If the test is to be read visually, then an enzyme and a substrate which produces a dense, easily visible colour is to be preferred. In that context horseradish peroxidase is difficult to better. Many substrates are available, ranging from the blue products of o-tolidine through the greens of 2,2′-azino-di[3-ethylbenzthiozoline sulfonate(6)] (ABTS) to the other end of the spectrum and the red-orange of o-phenylenediamine as well as the black of aminosalicylic acid. This article is not the place to discuss their individual merits; it suffices to say that of the numerous peroxidase substrates there are many suitable for both visual reading and by assessment with photometers.

For some purposes it may be preferable to detect the enzyme by means of a fluorescent substrate. In that case β-galactosidase or alkaline phosphatase may be used together with methyl umbelliferryl galactoside or phosphate (Ishikawa and Kato, 1978; Arakawa et al., 1983). Because of the sensitivity of fluorescence detection it is possible to miniaturize the assays so that very small amounts of reagents are used, but the tests are not necessarily sensitive in terms of analyte detection.

Recently, glucose 6-phosphate dehydrogenase has been used as a label in a sensitive fluorometric assay for haptens based on the measurement of reduced pyridine nucleotide (Shah et al., 1984). Enzymes have also been used as labels in conjunction with chemiluminescent substrates, and sensitive methods have been reported for the measurement of dehydroepiandrosterone (Arakawa et al., 1981) and 17α-hydroxyprogesterone (Arakawa et al., 1982). A procedure for enzyme-enhanced chemiluminescence immunoassay has been reported by Whitehead et al. (1983), and the reaction may be monitored with a photographic film (Thorpe et al., 1984).

As mentioned earlier, the other main component of ELISA, in addition to the enzyme conjugate, is the solid phase, to which the immuno-reagent is attached. The great virtue of using a solid phase-immobilized reagent is that it ¡permits very easy washing, replacing the tiresome centrifugation previously used in the second antibody precipitation methods. The most popular types of solid phases are those made of plastic moulded into tubes, beads, discs, pegs or, most common of all, into microplates which permit easy batch processing. Usually the antibody or antigen is passively adsorbed to the surface of the solid carrier material. This method has often been criticised but to date none of the claimed covalent methods of linkage have proved reliable. Unfortunately plastics show considerable variations in their ability to take up immuno-reagents and this property is dependent not only on the composition of the plastic, but also on its processing at the production stage. In general the aim is to achieve a high level of reproducible coating with the immunoreagent then minimal uptake of the sample and conjugate. The latter can be reduced by post-coating of the immuno-sensitized solid phase with irrelevant blocking protein (e.g. bovine serum albumin; BSA) and by the inclusion of wetting agents (e.g. Tween) with or without additional protein (e.g. BSA) into the diluent solutions. The combination of these treatments in most instances reduces the non-specific absorption to negligible proportions. Notwithstanding comments to the contrary it is possible to establish ELISA tests for proteins (e.g. α-fetoprotein, hCG) with similar sensitivity ($\cong 1$ ng ml^{-1}) and intra-assay precision (e.g. coefficients of variation of 8–10%) as can be achieved by RIA. In addition, ultrasensitive EIAs have been reported for the measurement of free thyroxine in serum (Ito et al., 1984) and progesterone in saliva (Tallon et al., 1984).Most of the problems reported by those investigators newly taking up EIA can be traced to inadequate quality assurance of the solid phase carriers, poor conjugates and lack of care in the washing steps. Those interested in setting up their own EIA systems should consult the technical reviews (Engvall and Pesce, 1978; Voller et al., 1979; Malvano, 1980; Avrameas et al., 1983; Voller and Bidwell, 1983, Blake and Gould, 1984).

ELISA has been used so extensively in recent years that it is of little value to give individual references. There have, however, been some useful reviews of the technique in the study of infectious diseases (Voller et al., 1979; Voller and Bidwell, 1980; Yolken, 1982), tumour-associated antigens (Masseyeff, 1978), veterinary medicine (Wardley and Crowther, 1982) and agriculture (Clark, 1981). It seems likely that eventually ELISA will be replaced by chemiluminescent- and fluorescent-labelled reagent methods where the highest sensitivity is required. However, the visual reading possibilities will ensure its continuance into the future as a rather simple field test, and the variety of available end-points will enable the methods to be presented in different formats.

REFERENCES

Arakawa, H., Maeda, M., Tsuji, A. and Kambegawa, A. (1981). Chemiluminescence enzyme immunoassay of dehydroepiandrosterone and its sulphate using peroxidase as label. *Steroids*, **38**, 453–464.

Arakawa, H., Maeda, M. and Tsuji, A. (1982). Chemiluminescence enzyme immunoassay of 17α-hydroxyprogesterone using glucose oxidase and bis(2,4,6-trichlorophenyl) oxalate–fluorescent dye system. *Chem. Pharm. Bull.* **30**, 3036–3039.

Arakawa, H., Maeda, M., Tsuji, A., Natuse, H., Suzuki, E. and Kambegawa, A. (1983). Fluorescence enzyme immunoassay of 17α-hydroxyprogesterone in dried blood samples on filter paper and its application to mass screening for congenital adrenal hyperplasia. *Chem. Pharm. Bull.* **31**, 2724–2731.

Avrameas, S., Druet, P., Masseyeff, R. and Feldman, G. (1983). Developments in immunology. In *Immunoenzymatic Techniques*, Vol. 18, Elsevier, Amsterdam, pp. 1–410.

Blake, C. and Gould, B. J. (1984). Use of enzymes in immunoassay techniques. A review. *Analyst* **109**, 533–547.

Clark, M. F. (1981). Immunosorbent assays in plant pathology. *A. Rev. Phytopath.* **19**, 83–106.

Curtiss, E. G. and Patel, J. A. (1978). Enzyme multiplied immunoassay techniques: a review. *CRC Crit. Rev. Clin. Lab. Sci.* **9**, 303–318.

Engvall, E. and Perlmann, P. (1971). Enzyme linked immunosorbent assay (ELISA): quantitative assay of IgG. *Immunochemistry* **8**, 871–874.

Engvall, E. and Pesce, A. J. (1978). Quantitative enzyme immunoassay. *Scand. J. Immunol.* **8** (Suppl. 7), 1–125.

Freytag, J. W., Dickinson, J. C. and Tseng, S. Y. (1984). A highly sensitive affinity-column-mediated immunometric assay, as exemplified by digoxin. *Clin. Chem.* **25**, 417–420.

Gibbons, I., Skold, C., Rowley, C. L. and Ullman, G. F. (1980). Homogeneous enzyme immunoassays for proteins employing β-galactosidase. *Analyt. Biochem.* **102**, 167–171.

Greenquist, A. C., Walter, B. and Li, T M. (1981). Homogeneous fluorescent immunoassay with dry reagents. *Clin. Chem.* **27**, 1614–1617.

Ishikawa, E. and Kato, K. (1978). Ultrasensitive enzyme immunoassay. *Scand. J. Immunol.* **8** (Suppl. 7), 43–55.

Ito, M., Miyai, K., Doi, K., Mizuta, H. and Amino, N. (1984). Enzyme immunoassay of free thyroxin in serum. *Clin. Chem.* **30**, 1682–1685.

Litman, D. J., Hanlon, T. M. and Ullman, E. F. (1980). Enzyme channelling immunoassay. *Analyt. Biochem.* **106**, 223–225.

Litman, D. J., Lee, R. H., Jeong, H. J., Tom, H. K., Stiso, S. N., Sizto, N. C. and Ullman, e. F. (1983). An internally referenced test strip immunoassay for morphine. *Clin. Chem.* **29**, 1598–1603.

Malvano, R. (1980). *Developments in Clinical Biochemistry*, Vol. 1, *Immunoenzymatic Assay Techniques*, Martinus Nijhoff, The Hague.

Masseyeff, r. (1978) Assay of tumour-associated antigens. *Scand. J. Immunol.* **8**, (Suppl. 7), 83–90.

Ngo, T. T., Carrico, R. J., Boggslaski, R. C. and Burd, J. F. (1981). Homogeneous substrate labelled fluorescent immunoassay for IgG in human serum. *J. Immunol. Meth.* **42**, 93–97.

Niewola, Z., Walsh, S. T. and Davies, G. E. (1983). Enzyme linked immunosorbent assay (ELISA) for paraquat. *Int. J. Immunopharmac.* **5**, 211–218.

Oellerich, M. (1980) Enzyme immunoassays in clinical chemistry. *J. Clin. Chem. Clin. Biochem.* **18**, 197–206.

Shah, H., Saranko, A. M., Harkonen, M. and Adlercreutz, H. (1984). Direct solid-phase fluoroenzyme immunoassay of 5β-pregnane-3α,20α-diol-3α-glucuronide in urine. *Clin. Chem.* **30**, 185–187.

Tallon, O. F., Gosling, J. P., Buckley, P. M., Dooley, M. H., Cleere, W. F., O'Dwyer, E. M. and Fottrell, P. F. (1984). Direct solid-phase enzyme immunoassay of progesterone in saliva. *Clin. Chem.* **30**, 1507–1511.

Thorpe, G. H. G., Whitehead, T. P., Penn, R. and Kricka, L. J. (1984). Photographic monitoring of enhanced luminescent immunoassays. *Clin. Chem.* **30**, 806–807.

Tyhach, R. J., Rupchock, P. A., Prendergrass, J. H., Skjold, A. C., Smith, P. J., Johnson, R. D., Albarella, J. P. and Profitt, J. A. (1981). Adaptation of prosthetic-group-label homogeneous immunoassay to reagent-strip format. *Clin. Chem.* **27**, 1499–1504.

Van Weemen, B. K. and Schuurs, A. H. W. M. (1972). Immunoassay using hapten–enzyme conjugates. *FEBS Lett.*, **24**, 77–81.

Voller, A. and Bidwell, D. E. (1980). *The Enzyme Linked Immunosorbent Assay*, Vol. 2. *A Review of Recent Developments with Abstracts of Microplate Applications*, MicroSystems, Guernsey.

Voller, A. & Bidwell, D. E. (1983). Heterogeneous enzyme immunoassays (ELISA)—difficulties encountered and their resolution. In *Biologie Prospective*, Masson, Paris, pp. 217–222.

Voller, A., Bidwell, D. E. and Bartlett, A. (1979). *The Enzyme Linked Immunosorbent Assay: A Guide with Abstracts of Microplate Applications*, Dynatech, Guernsey.

Wade, H. G., Danisch, R. J., Baxter, S. R., Federici, M. M., Fraser, R. C., Brownmiller, L. J. and Lankford, J. C. (1982) Enzyme immunoassay of the glycoprotein tropic hormones–HCG, lutropin, thyrotropin–with solid-phase monoclonal antibody for the α-subunit and enzyme coupled monoclonal antibody specific for the α-subunit. *Clin. Chem.* **28**, 1862–1866.

Wardley, R. C. and Crowther, J. R. (1982). The ELISA in veterinary research and diagnosis. *Curr. Top. Vet. Med. Anim. Sci.* **22**, 1–319.

Whitehead, T. P., Thorpe, G. H. G., Carter, T. J. N., Groucutt, C. and Kricka, L. J. (1983). Enhanced luminescence procedure for sensitive determination of peroxidase-labelled conjugates in immunoassay. *Nature, Lond.* **305**, 158–159.

Wong, R. C., Burd, J. F., Carrico, R. T., Thoma, J. and Boguslaski, R. C. (1979). Substrate-labelled fluorescent immunoassay for phenytoin in human serum. *Clin. Chem.* **25**, 686–688.

Yolken, R. H. (1982) Enzyme immunoassays for the detection of infectious agents in body fluids. *Rev. Infect. Dis.* **4**, 35–68.

CHAPTER 7

Instrumentation: photometric and photon emission immunoassays

E. SOINI

Wallac Oy,
PO Box 10,
20101 Turku 10,
Finland

1. INTRODUCTION

Non-isotopic immunoassays can be classified in many different ways. The nature of the *label* can be used for this purpose, and another more commonly used criterium is the *detection* method. In the field of non-isotopic immunoassays there are two major methods of detection based on the use of light: (i) photometric, and (ii) photon emission, i.e. chemiluminescence and delayed fluorescence. The purpose of this chapter is to present a critical study of photon emission methods and to make a comparative study of their performance and robustness.

2. PHOTOMETRIC METHODS

Many particle immunoassays and enzyme immunoassays belong to this category. The traditional immunoassay is based on haemagglutination, where the red blood cells are used as visual markers on a microtitre plate. Methods based on nephelometry and particle counting represent a more advanced version. Immunoassays with such detection methods are widely used today. Suitable instrumentation is available from a number of manufacturers. The use of nephelometry has been limited to serum protein assays (Gauldie,

1981). Particle counting, and especially latex particle counting, has been found useful not only for the measurement of serum proteins, but also for drug monitoring and some hormones analyses. The latex particle counting immunoassay is based on a laser instrument. The reagent is a suspension of latex particles coated with an antibody, antigen or hapten. The instrument counts the unagglutinated particles using an optical particle counter, and a change in the number of particles is inversely proportional to the concentration of the analyte (Cambiaso et al., 1977).

Conventional spectrophotometers and clinical analysers can be successfully used for various enzyme immunoassays. In this category we should also add the interesting dye sol immunoassay (see Chapter 4 in this volume), where colour formation as the result of agglutination can be measured with a photometer. There is a wide selection of dedicated photometers for enzyme immunoassays available today from various instrument manufacturers. The great problem in this field is the standardization of the measuring cuvette. The developments in this field have led to a situation where a variety of special cuvettes have been developed, but cuvettes based on the multiwell ('microtitre', 'microwell') plates seem to be used increasingly. Multiwell plates and strips are very useful and are well accepted as a standard in the immunoassay field. However, they involve a technical challenge for photometric detection in high performance immunoassays. The sensitivity at the low concentration end of the absorbance scale is not yet very satisfactory. Improved sensitivity and precision require multiwell plates with high optical quality and uniformity between the wells. Scratches or cloudiness in the plastic material increase the scattering of the photometric light beam and cause variation in the results. This limitation is naturally a problem in nephelometry as well. Another problem in photometric detection is the limited dynamic concentration range. This aspect requires careful optimization of the assay composition so that the dynamic range of the instrument fits the relevant clinical concentration range of the analyte.

3.   PHOTON EMISSION TECHNIQUES

By true photon emission techniques we mean chemiluminometry and time-resolved fluorometry involving the unique advantage of the emission signal being physically separated from excitation. In chemiluminometry the separation is the result of chemical excitation and physical emission. In time-resolved fluorometry the excitation and emission are separated by a time delay.

A unique advantage of photon emission techniques is the extremely high specific activity of the label in terms of emitted photons per second. This property is due to the fact that the excited states of the chemiluminescent or fluorescent probes are created in the measuring position of the sample. The emission rate is a function of the excitation intensity and decay time.

Fluorescent probes are even more favourable because the excitation can be increased by the higher intensity of the exciting radiation, whereas chemiluminescence excitation has certain practical limitations. The optimal decay time of fluorescent probes for the time-resolved fluorometry is 10–1000 μs. The decay time of chemiluminescence probes typically ranges from 1 to 20 s. There is a tendency to develop chemiluminescent probes of a longer decay time to simplify the luminometric measurement. This modification is, however, done at the cost of the specific activity. A typical specific activity of photon emission probes reaches up to 10^7 photon s^{-1} for 1 pmol of the labelled compound. For useful radioisotopic labels the specific activity does not exceed 10^3 disintegration s^{-1} for 1 pmol of the labelled compound.

Another important advantage of the photon emission techniques is the wide dynamic range. In luminometry and fluorometry the dynamic range of the instrument is typically five decades of linear scale. This can be exploited successfully in immunometric assays for certain analytes (hCG, TSH, AFP, HBsAg) which require a very wide dynamic range. Photon emission techniques, including chemiluminescence and fluorescence, have the important advantage over photometric assays of not being too dependent on the optical quality of the cuvette. Photons detected are not from the collimated light beam as in photometers and the scattering plays a much more minor role. As a consequence, photon emission techniques have an extremely high sensitivity. They provide a very high count rate with a low instrument background. In chemiluminometry and time-resolved fluorometry concentrations down to 10^{-17} mol per cuvette can be detected. It is important to realize that the limiting factor for the lowest level of detection in a practical immunoassay is not the instrument background or signal to noise ratio, but the signal from the blank sample. In luminometry the non-specific chemiluminescence reactions play an important role. In time-resolved fluorometry the background is determined in practice only by the non-specific binding effects.

4. LUMINESCENCE

A number of chemiluminescence immunoassays (CIAs) have been presented in the literature: (i) CIA with cofactor label (ATP, NADH) and bioluminescence detection; (ii) CIA with an isoluminol label and chemiluminescence detection; (iii) CIA with cofactor producing enzyme label and bioluminescence detection; (iv) CIA with microperoxidase label and chemiluminescence detection. Most of these chemiluminescence immunoassays involve the use of enzymes as labels. They naturally also involve similar chemical problems to enzyme immunoassays in general, including stereochemical effects and proteolysis etc.

A basic luminometer is a very simple instrument in principle. The detector block comprises only the measuring chamber and a photon detector. For this reason, a luminometer is potentially a very inexpensive instrument. Present chemistry, however, sets certain special requirements on the instrument, which makes the current automatic luminometers quite complex and expensive. In this context the injection of the activator reagent and mixing could be mentioned. The functional principle and design concept of the LKB–Wallac automatic Luminometer 1251 appear in Figs 1, 2 and 3. The instrument comprises fully automated functions and data reduction, a sample magazine for 25 samples, a high precision thermostat ($\pm$ 0.1 °C) for samples and the detector, and an option for injection and mixing. This instrument was originally made for kinetic enzyme assays, but is very useful in CIA as well. Special attention should be paid to the complexity of functions required in a number of multi-purpose luminometers, and especially to the detector block of the 1251, which has been designed in a very elegant way. Many necessary physical functions have been neatly incorporated in the same compact module:

(i) a highly sensitive photon counter
(ii) a sample magazine

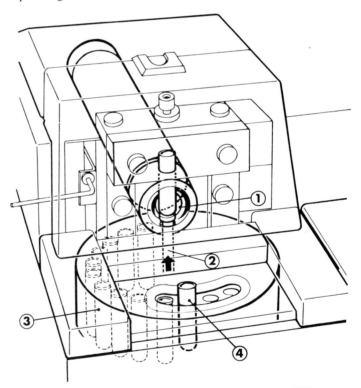

Fig. 1. Functional principle of the LKB–Wallac Luminometer 1251. 1, measuring chamber with light reflector; 2, elevator; 3, sample carousel; 4, sample loading position

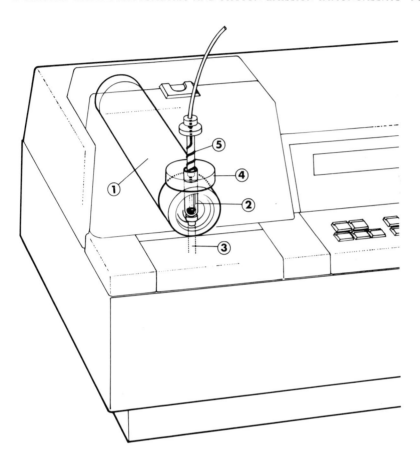

Fig. 2. Functional principle of the LKB–Wallac Luminometer 1251. 1, photomultiplier tube; 2, sample cuvette (LKB 2174–086) with special inside wings for proper mixing; 3, elevator; 4, mixing device including electric motor; 5, reagent injection tubings: spiral-formed feedthrough for three tubings and a straight feedthrough for one thin steel needle (only one tubing illustrated)

  (iii) a precision thermostat and thermal isolation
  (iv) a sample elevator
   (v) a light-tight measuring chamber
  (vi) a splash-free and drop-free reagent injection
 (vii) an option for one, two or three reagent injection needles and dispensers
(viii) mixing
  (ix) a quick release and easy-to-clean measuring chamber, with a quick visual inspection of the injection needles.

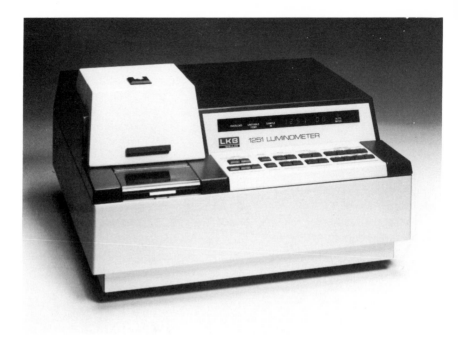

Fig. 3. LKB–Wallac Luminometer 1251

The activator reagent injection is crucial for high precision. The 1251 luminometer can be equipped with automatic dispensers (Model 1291), which provide a rapid adjustable volume reagent injection (Model 1291–100) between 5 μl and 35 μl or between 10 μl and 350 μl (Model 1291–101). The dispenser is based on the peristaltic pumping principle, as shown in Figs 4 and 5. The precision is better than 0.5% for volumes over 10 μl.

The reaction conditions of the luminescence emission after the injection, besides the chemical conditions, are affected by the speed and volume of the injection as well as on the mixing. Mixing is necessary for small injection volumes, but for larger volumes over 200 μl mixing is carried out by turbulence caused by rapid injection. Typical luminescence kinetics are shown, for example, in a paper by Pazzagli et al. (1981). Integration of the signal up to 20–30 s is also important for improved precision.

General requirements for a CIA luminometer are listed below:

(i) an automatic sample changer
(ii) a dispenser for at least one and preferably three reagents at measuring position

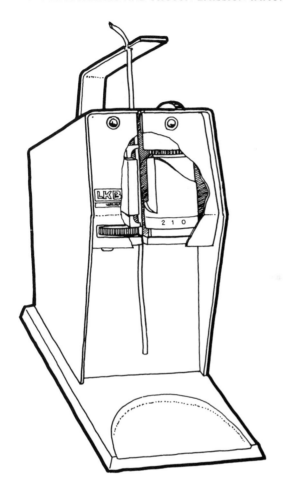

Fig. 4. Design concept of the LKB–Wallac Automatic Dispenser 1291

(iii) a method of mixing–not necessary if activator injection volume and speed are high enough
(iv) an integration of the signal response up to 30 s
(v) a sensitivity requirement, S/N = 1 for 10^{-12} mol^{-1} ATP with the firefly luciferase system as calibrated with the LKB–Wallac ATP Monitoring reagent
(vi) a detector and sample at room temperature ± 1°C.

The sensitivity is given in units of ATP, because so far it is the only useful and commonly relevant standard. The absolute photon standards are not avail-

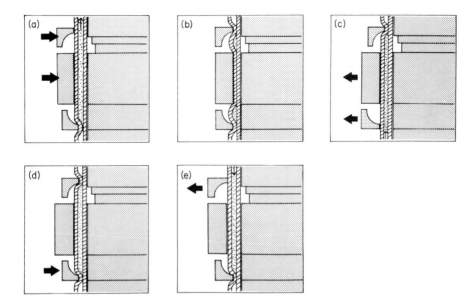

Fig. 5. The functional principle of the LKB-Wallac Dispenser 1291. The arrows indicate the direction of the movement. The dispenser mechanism comprises a pressure bar and two valve bars which produce reproducible squeezing action against the flat side of a metal cylinder. The silicon capillary tube through which the liquid is dispensed is fitted between the pressure bar and the side of the cylinder. When the cylinder is rotated, a different width of metal is exposed to the pressure bar which in turn means that a different length of capillary tube is squeezed and the adjustable volume control is achieved. Step-by-step action is as follows: (a) pumping action; (b) after dispensing the valves are closed; (c) the capillary is refilled; (d) when the capillary is full the inlet valve is closed; (e) the outlet valve is opened before the liquid is dispensed

able yet. We have, however, started a programme for developing such standards.

The main problem in CIA is the reproducibility, which may be affected by the varying background, and interference from the biological sample. A satisfactory methodology and ideal reagents are still anticipated (see Chapters 8 and 9 of this volume). The results of Whitehead et al. (1983) on enzyme-enhanced chemiluminescence immunoassay are very encouraging because the exploitation of the constant light signal and high intensity luminescence system considerably simplifies the instrument requirements. The reagent injection would no longer be a critical step and mixing would be completely eliminated.

Luminometry in general has a very wide linear dynamic range which, with analogue detectors, at best covers five to six decades. In a practical immunochemiluminometric assay the linearity of the instrument has not been exploited, because the signal response of the luminescence is not linear with the analyte concentration. The immunoreaction itself creates an inhibition effect, the nature of which is not yet understood.

4.1. Conventional fluorometry

Fluoroimmunoassays (FIAs), which are based on conventional fluorometry involving the use of organic fluorescent probes with short-lived fluorescence, such as fluorescein isothiocyanate (FITC) and rhodamines include (i) FIA with FITC-label (heterogeneous); (ii) polarization FIA (homogeneous); (iii) quenching FIA (homogeneous), and (iv) FIA with enzyme label and fluorescent substrate or product.

Conventional fluorometry suffers from several problems: separation of fluorescence emission from excitation; Rayleigh scattering; Raman scattering; background fluorescence (cuvette and optics; fluorescence in the sample blank, e.g. serum; free fluorescent probes); effects due to too high excitation intensity (photodecomposition (irreversible); bleaching (reversible)); background of photodetector (thermal noise); fluorescence quenching (chemical quenching; concentration quenching; self-absorption).

It is apparent from the excitation and emission spectra of fluorescein (Fig. 6) and especially the overlapping of the spectra and the autofluorescence of the compounds of blood serum (Fig. 7), that conventional fluorescence has a minor potential in immunoassays for analytes in serum samples. Even assays involving solid phase separation and washing steps suffer from background signal from the cuvette. An interesting approach to reduce the plastic cuvette background signal has been introduced by Dynatec. The 'Microfluor' fluorometer uses black-coloured microtitre strips and the manufacturer claims that the background is reduced significantly.

Due to the problems discussed above, fluorometry has not been extensively used in immunology. A high and varying background is present except in the measurement of high concentration analytes, such as serum proteins and drugs. Enzymatic amplification (Wong et al., 1979) has considerably improved the sensitivity, but it involves a relatively complex chemical system with an increased demand for quality control at the cost of robustness. The polarization FIA (Dandliker and de Soussure, 1970; Dandliker et al., 1973; Spencer, 1981) and quenching and transfer FIA (Ullman et al., 1976) offer very simple and straightforward assay procedures. They have been found useful and are widely accepted in certain fields. However, the applicability is limited not only by the low sensitivity, but also by the very narrow dynamic range. The limited dynamic range is produced by the combination of two non-linear processes: (i) competitive binding versus analyte concentration and (ii) polarization change measure versus complex formation. The dynamic range is hardly wider than one decade. In addition, the polarization FIA is

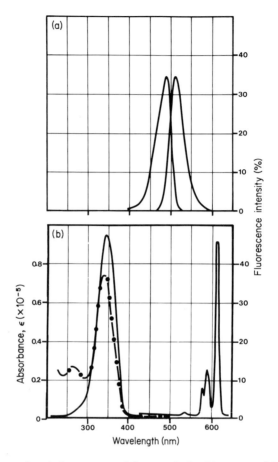

Fig. 6. Excitation and emission spectra of fluorescein isothiocyanate (a) and europium (b). ———, excitation and emission; ●—●, absorption

useful only for the measurement of small-size antigens. The varying background has been improved by employing the test slide technology (Kronick and Little, 1975; Harte, 1981), which in combination with a washing step significantly improves the quality of FIA.

4.2. Time-resolved fluorometry

Chelates of europium and terbium are potential alternatives to radioisotopic and other non-isotopic labels in immunoassays. Many lanthanides are fluorescent and have been exploited in various fields (e.g. electroluminescence and

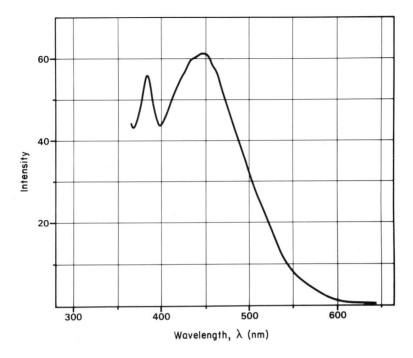

Fig. 7. Fluorescence emission of blood serum for excitation at 340 nm

lasers). The main advantages of using chelates as fluorescent probes are the high quantum yield, exceptionally large Stokes' shift, narrow emission peaks, and optimal emission and excitation wavelength for use with biological material (cf. Figs 6 and 7). These characteristics make the lanthanide chelates preferable to conventional fluorescent probes even for use with ordinary fluorometers.

Because of the natural fluorescence from various compounds such as serum proteins in biological samples, the conventional fluorescent probes suffer from serious limitations of sensitivity. With lanthanide chelates, however, it is possible to reduce the background level considerably by the selective detection of long-decay fluorescence. The fluorescence decay time of lanthanide chelates is often of the order of 10–100 μs, whereas the corresponding time of natural fluorescence in a typical biological sample is in the order of 1–20 ns. For this reason, the pulsed-light source, time-resolved fluorometers used in conjunction with lanthanide chelates are potentially several orders of magnitude more sensitive than conventional fluorometers (Soini and Hemmilä, 1979).

Studies on time-resolved fluoroimmunoassay were started in our laboratory in 1974. The potential use of lanthanides soon became clear when it was realized that even the most favourable organic fluorescent probes have a fluorescence decay time of less than 100 ns, which required very sophisticated and expensive instrumentation. Towards the end of the 1970s the concept of using lanthanides as fluorescent probes was made practical and viable in co-operation with a number of collaborating laboratories. In this programme the contribution of Professor R. Ekins has been considerable, especially in guiding our research strategy in the immunoassay field towards more sensitive immunoassays, and in pointing out the great potential in the combination of the labelled antibody technique and time-resolved fluorescence.

Originally we developed a simple, manually operated fluorometer for fluoroimmunoassays with lanthanide chelates. Seven units, as shown in the block diagram in Fig. 8, were produced for research purposes only. The

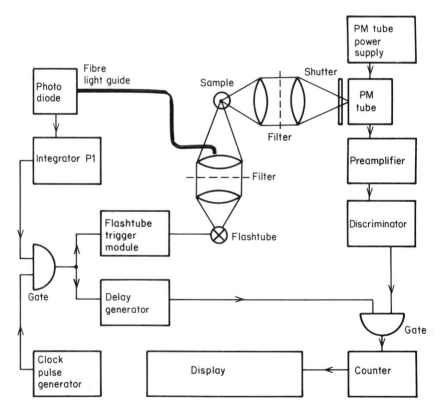

Fig. 8. The functional block diagram of the time-resolved fluorometer

sample compartment is covered by a light-tight lid and the sample is changed manually. The reaction mixtures are held in small disposable tubes or cuvettes made of polystyrene which has a reasonably low long-decay background fluorescence. The pulsed light source in this fluorometer is a xenon flashtube equipped with a suitable interference filter for an excitation band. Because the intensity of the single flashes from the xenon flashtube was not sufficiently reproducible, we had to ensure stabilization of the excitation system. An integrator (P1) for a semiconductor photodiode serves as the stabilizer of the flashlamp. The flashlamp is activated about 10^3 times at a frequency of 1 kHz. The exact number of flashes (N) is controlled by the integrator P1 so that the integrated intensity of the photon emission is fixed. As the stabilization detector we used a photodiode connected to the optical system by a fibre light guide. The integrated photon emission from the flashtube is stabilized by this method with a precision of $\pm(1/N)\times100\%$ assuming that the deviation of the intensity of single flashes is not greater than $\pm50\%$.

This stabilization method has many advantages. First of all, the system is simple; the flashtube and its power supply can be made without a stabilization circuit, and less expensive flashtubes with lower stability can be used. The temperature dependence of the system can be minimized by a single compensator element. The flashtube is operated only during measurement, thus ensuring a long practical life. The eventual fatigue of the flashtube will be automatically compensated for by the integrator. The photomultiplier tube, operated in the single-photon mode, is connected to a fast preamplifier and discriminator and a fast scaler which has a digital display of seven decades. The counting speed of random events is limited to 40 MHz by the preamplifier and single-photon discriminator. Figure 9 shows a commercially available unit, which is substantially similar in design.

In parallel with the fluorometer development, the efforts in our laboratory were directed to synthesizing a stable fluorescent chelate for use as a label in time-resolved fluoroimmunoassay or immunofluorometric assay. A suitable fluorescent europium (Eu) chelate would be combination of EDTA-Eu-β-NTA, where the EDTA serves as a suitable complexing means for labelling the antibody and β-NTA (2-naphthoyltrifluoroacetone) makes the lanthanide fluorescent (Soini and Hemmilä, 1979). This structure can, however, be mentioned only as an example of a hypothetical fluorescent probe for the time-resolved fluoroimmunoassay (TR-FIA). The combination is not stable and the fluorescence is extinguished by water. A practical solution for a stable lanthanide label and stable fluorescence detection was developed in 1979. In this approach the lanthanide was bound to the antibody by using an aminophenyl derivative of EDTA. The amino group was activated by diazotization and then reacted with tyrosine and histidine residues in the protein to be labelled. The conjugation reaction produced a stable complex

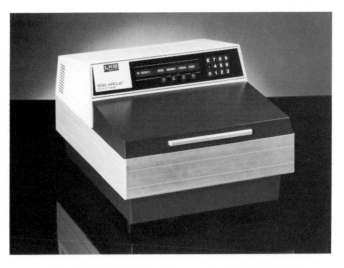

Fig. 9. LKB–Wallac fluorometer 1230 'ARCUS'

which is used in the immunoassay. This complex is, however, non-fluorescent-virtually a metal label. The measurement of labelled antigen–antibody conjugates was carried out after separation, by adding another chelating agent–in an enhancement solution, which dissociates the europium ion from the antibody–chelate complex and forms a β-NTA chelate creating an intense fluorescence with europium. A synergistic agent of trioctylphosphine oxide further enhances the fluorescence of the chelate (Hemmilä et al., 1984).

The coated tube technology has been used in practical immunoassays and the Eu-EDTA-labelled antibody reacted with an immobilized antigen on the solid phase. The fluorescent chelate was formed in the solution after dissociation of the Eu ion. This configuration presents a significant advantage from the fluorometric point of view. The detection of the fluorescence signal in solution is much more stable and reproducible than in the solid phase. The signal is not dependent on the homogeneity of the coating nor on the position of the tube in the fluorometer detector. The photon collection geometry is also better, and the tube makes only a minor contribution to the background signal. The addition of the enhancement solution naturally involves an extra step in the assay procedure, but the formation of the fluorescent chelate is rapid and equilibrium is achieved in a few minutes.

The present methodology is simple and straightforward for immunoassays which require high performance. It is highly insensitive to interferences from the sample because the methodology involves three steps to minimize the problem: (i) washing, which cleans the cuvette of interfering constituents in the sample; (ii) dissociation of the biochemically inert Eu ion from the solid phase and formation of a new chelate, which provides a stable and reproducible fluorescence, and (iii) the time-resolved fluorescence detection eliminates the autofluorescence of the materials in the system, as well as the possible interfering residues from the sample.

The present methodology called DELFIA ('dissociation-enhanced lanthanide fluoroimmunoassay') has been developed for a number of analytes including hCG, TSH, HBsAg, AFP, certain steroids and viral antigens. The methods have been found to be simple and robust for routine clinical use.

5. EVALUATION OF PHOTON EMISSION IMMUNOASSAYS

Certain important performance parameters of photon emission immunoassays are summarized below and compared with those of photometric methods including enzyme immunoassay. The common important performance limiting factors are the non-specific binding effects and the sample preparation error which are not discussed in this context. The photon emission methods in general and time-resolved fluorometry in particular, offer an extraordinarily wide *dynamic range* $(1 : 10^4)$ and linearity which cover the whole concentration range of clinical importance without extra dilution of the sample. The large linearity can be exploited only in the immunometric assays because the competitive binding assay principle works only on a very limited dynamic range. The dynamic range of the photometric methods is limited by the principle of photometry and in practice does not exceed 1:100. Methods based on inhibition, quenching or fluorescence polarization also have a very limited dynamic range. The need for *sensitivity* in terms of the detection limit is to be assessed for each analyte separately. A generally applicable method, however, should have the highest possible sensitivity, and photon emission methods fulfil this requirement in a more trouble-free way than photometric methods. The extra step of the *procedure*, which involves either the activator reagent injection (chemiluminometry) or addition of the enhancement reagent (TR-FIA), is a disadvantage. The enhancement reaction is, however, very rapid and trouble-free and presents undoubtedly a lesser complication than the activation of the enzyme reaction in the photometric methods. The more linear the dose–response curve, the simpler is the *standardization* of the assay. In this respect time-resolved fluorometry is superior to any photometric method. Good *intra-assay precision* can be achieved with many different immunoassay methods. In photometric methods the quality of cuvettes should be controlled very carefully, whereas in photon emission methods quality errors which increase the scattered light emission are not important. Enzymes offer one unique advantage–the colour formation–and are therefore very useful in qualitative visual reading immunoassays in decentralized diagnostics. On the basis of the features presented above, photon emission techniques have the potential to become the most widely used methods in high performance routine immunoassays, and may be automated for use in centralized diagnostics.

REFERENCES

Cambiaso, C. L., Leek, A. E., De Steenwinkel, F., Billen, J. and Masson, P. L. (1977). Particle counting immunoassay (PACIA). I. A general method for the determination of antibodies, antigens and haptens. *J. Immunol. Meth.* **18**, 33–44.

Dandliker, W. B. and de Saussure, V. A. (1970). Fluorescence polarization in immunochemistry. *Immunochemistry* **7**, 799–828.

Dandliker, W. B., Kelly, R. J. and Dandliker, J. (1973). Fluorescence polarization immunoassay. Theory and experimental method. *Immunochemistry*, **10**, 219–227.

Dandliker, W. B. *et al.*, (1978). Fluorescence methods for measuring reaction equilibria and kinetics. *Meth. Enzymol.* **48**, 380–414.

Gauldie, J. (1981). Principles and clinical applications of nephelometry. In *Nonisotopic Alternatives to Radioimmunoassay* (L. A. Kaplan and A. J. Pesce, eds), Marcel Dekker, New York, pp. 285–322.

Harte, R. A. (1981). Fluoroimmunometry and the FIAX system. In *Nonisotopic Alternatives to Radioimmunoassay* (L. A. Kaplan and A. J. Pesce, eds), Marcel Dekker, New York, pp. 285–322.

Hemmilä, I., Dakubu, S., Mukkala, V.-M., Siitari, H. and Lövgren, T. (1984). Europium as a label in time-resolved immunofluorometric assays. *Analyt. Biochem.* **137**, 335–343.

Kronick, M. N. and Little, W. A. (1975). A new immunoassay based on fluorescence excitation by internal reflection spectroscopy. *J. Immunol. Meth.* **8**, 235–240.

Kronick, M. N. and Little, W. A. (1976). Fluorescent immunoassay employing total reflection for activation. US Patent no. 3,939,350.

Pazzagli, M., Kim, J. B., Messeri, G., Kohen, F., Bolelli, G. F., Tommasi, A., Salerno, R. and Serio, M. (1981). Luminescent immunoassay (LIA) of cortisol-2. Development and validation of the immunoassay monitored by chemiluminescence. *J. Steroid Biochem.* **14**, 1181–1187.

Soini, E. and Hemmilä, I. (1979). Fluoroimmunoassay: present status and key problems. *Clin. Chem.* **25**, 353–361.

Spencer, R. D. (1981). Applications of fluorescent polarization in clinical assays. In *Nonisotopic Alternatives to Radioimmunoassay* (L. A. Kaplan and A. J. Pesce, eds), Marcel Dekker, New York, pp. 143–170.

Ullman, E. F., Schwartzberg, M. and Rubenstein, K. D. (1976). Fluorescent excitation transfer assay–a general method for determination of antigen. *J. Biol. Chem.* **251**, 4172–4178.

Whitehead, T. P., Thorpe, G. H. G., Carter, T. J. N., Groucott, C. and Kricka, L. T. (1983). Enhanced luminescence procedure for sensitive determination of peroxidase-labelled conjugates in immunoassay. *Nature, Lond.* **305**, 158–159.

Wong, R. C., Burd, R. F., Carrico, R. J., Buckler, R. T., Thoma, J. and Boguslaski, R. C. (1979). Substrate-labelled fluorescent immunoassay for phenytoin in human serum. *Clin. Chem.* **25**, 686–688.

CHAPTER 8

Chemiluminescence and bioluminescence immunoassay

F. Kohen,† M. Pazzagli,‡ M. Serio,‡ J. de Boever§ and D. Vandekerckhove§

† Department of Hormone Research,
The Weitzmann Institute of Science,
Rehovot, Israel

‡ Institute of Endocrinology,
University of Florence,
Florence, Italy

and

§ Department of Obstetrics and Gynaecology,
Academic Hospital,
Gent, Belgium

1. INTRODUCTION

Radioimmunoassay (RIA) is widely used for the determination of a variety of substances such as hormones, drugs and steroid metabolites in biological fluids. Although RIA procedures offer significant advantages over previously existing methods in terms of specificity and sensitivity, they depend on the availability of a suitable radiolabelled ligand. Furthermore, the dependence of RIA on radioactive labels has raised several problems which include: (i) the shelf-life and stability of radiolabelled compounds; (ii) the disposal of radioactive waste, and (iii) the relatively high cost of counting equipment needed for the end-point determination.

Recent studies from our laboratory (Kohen *et al.*, 1979, 1980a, 1981a, 1982, 1983; Barnard *et al.*, 1981a,b; Lindner *et al.*, 1981; Pazzagli *et al.*, 1981a,b,c,d; Eshhar *et al.*, 1981; Kim *et al.*, 1982; Weerasekera *et al.*, 1982; Kohen and Lindner, 1983; Collins *et al.*, 1983) and elsewhere (Pratt *et al.*, 1978; Schroeder *et al.*, 1976a,b, 1977, 1978, 1979; Maier, 1977, 1978; Shroeder and Yeager, 1978; Wannlund and DeLuca, 1981; Wannlund *et al.*,

1980; Weeks *et al.*, 1983a,b) have shown that chemiluminescence immunoassay can be a feasible alternative to RIA since luminescent tagged conjugates have been shown to be stable, and analytes can be measured at the level of pmol $\ell^{-}1$ (Pazzagli *et al.*, 1981b,c; Weeks *et al.*, 1983a). We report here the use of luminescent substances as labels in immunoassay, and the development of chemiluminescence- and bioluminescence-based immunoassays.

2. CLASSIFICATION OF LUMINESCENT IMMUNOASSAYS

Luminescent substances such as chemi- or bioluminescent molecules have been used in immunological reactions either directly as labels or indirectly in the quantitation by luminescence of enzyme or co-factor labelled antigens or antibodies. Based on these applications, the following types of luminescent immunoassays have emerged, as illustrated in Fig. 1:

$$Ag + Ag - L + Ab \rightleftharpoons Ab : Ag + Ab : Ag - L$$

Fig. 2. Principle of luminescent immunoassay. L = chemi or bioluminescent molecule, a cofactor, or an enzyme.

   (i) *Chemiluminescence immunoassay*   In this type of assay the antigen is tagged with a chemiluminescent molecule, such as isoluminol or acridinium ester, which emits light in a high quantum yield upon oxidation (Fig. 1, L = chemiluminescent molecule).

  (ii) *Bioluminescence immunoassay*   In this method the antigen is labelled with a bioluminescent substance such as luciferin (Fig. 1, L = bioluminescent molecule) or with a co-factor [nicotinamide adenine dinucleotide (NAD) or adenosine-5'-triphosphate (ATP)], which will participate directly or indirectly in a luminescent reaction (Fig. 1, L = co-factor). The latter type has been classified by Kricka and Carter (1982) as 'luminescent co-factor immunoassay'.

 (iii) *Chemiluminescent enzyme immunoassay*   In this type of assay the antigen is labelled with an enzyme (Fig. 1, L = enzyme) such as horseradish peroxidase (see Chapter 6 in this volume). At the end of the immunological reaction the enzyme is detected by chemiluminescence with luminol/luciferin/hydrogen peroxide (Whitehead *et al.*, 1983) more sensitively than by colorimetry.

In this chapter we will review the development of chemiluminescence- and bioluminescence-based immunoassays for haptens extracted from plasma, and for their metabolites in diluted urine.

3. CHEMILUMINESCENCE IMMUNOASSAYS

To date, luminol- or isoluminol-based chemiluminescence forms the basis of this type of immunoassay. The oxidation of luminol under basic conditions in the presence of a catalyst (e.g. microperoxidase) and hydrogen peroxide yields 3-aminophthalate and a high quantum yield of light (Fig. 2). Substitution of the aromatic amino group of luminol impairs its light-producing properties. In contrast, substitution of the aromatic amino group of isoluminol by alkyl chains enhances the light output (Schroeder and Yaeger, 1978; Schroeder et al., 1978). The use of primary amino derivatives of isoluminol as labels to monitor specific protein-binding reactions has been reported for biotin (Schroeder et al., 1976b) and for thyroxine (Schroeder et al., 1977). Since these derivatives can be measured at the pmol $\ell^{-}1$ level (Schroeder and Yeager, 1978), we used them as markers for covalent attachment to carboxy derivatives of steroids or urinary steroid glucuronides.

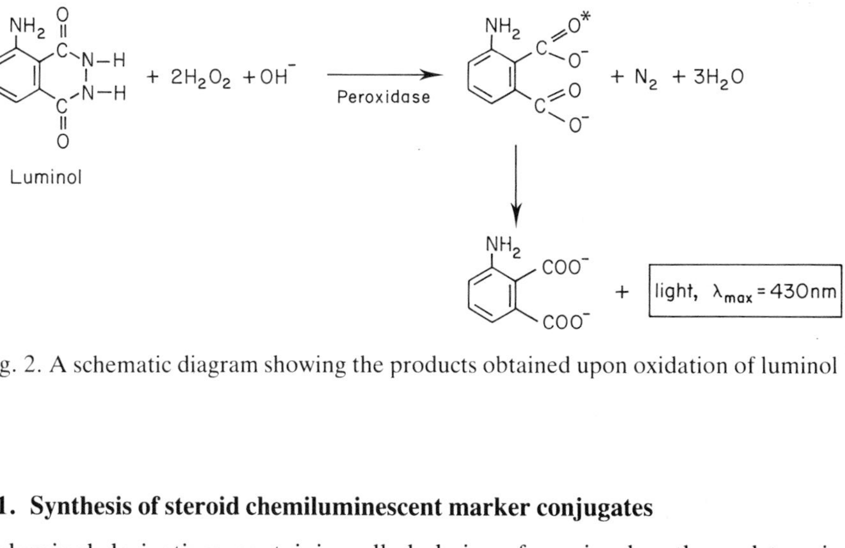

Fig. 2. A schematic diagram showing the products obtained upon oxidation of luminol

3.1. Synthesis of steroid chemiluminescent marker conjugates

Isoluminol derivatives containing alkyl chains of varying lengths and terminating with primary amino groups have been synthesized according to Schroeder et al. (1978). These compounds belong to the 6-[N-(α-aminoalkyl)-N-ethyl]-amino-2,3-dihydro-1,4-phtalazine-1,4-dione series and contain a bridging group of two methylene groups (aminoethylethylisoluminol, AEEI; Fig. 3, $n = 2$); four methylene groups (aminobutylethylisoluminol, ABEI; Fig. 3, $n = 4$), five methylene groups (aminopentylethylisoluminol, APEI; Fig. 3, $n = 5$) or six methylene groups (aminohexylethylisoluminol, AHEI; Fig. 3, $n = 6$).

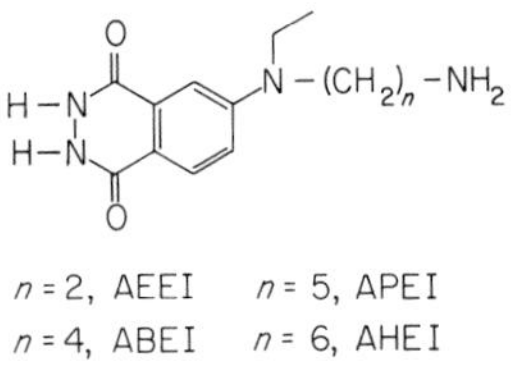

$$n = 2, \text{AEEI} \qquad n = 5, \text{APEI}$$
$$n = 4, \text{ABEI} \qquad n = 6, \text{AHEI}$$

Fig. 3. Structures of primary amino derivatives of isoluminol

The steroid–chemiluminescent marker conjugates were prepared in two steps: (i) a carboxy derivative of a steroid or a steroid glucuronide was activated in the presence of carbodiimide and N-hydroxysuccinimide to an activated ester; (ii) the activated steroid ester derivative was reacted with the primary amino group of an isoluminol derivative at basic pH to form a stable peptide bond (Fig. 4). The conjugates were purified by thin-layer chromatography (Pazzagli *et al.*, 1981a,c) and characterized by ultraviolet spectroscopy and mass spectrometry (Pazzagli *et al.*, 1983). When tested in a charcoal radioimmunoassay system each conjugate exhibited a binding affinity similar to the unaltered hapten (Pazzagli *et al.*, 1981c).

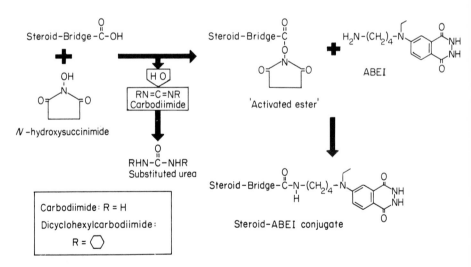

Fig. 4. A general synthetic scheme for the preparation of a chemiluminescent marker-steroid conjugate

3.2. Measurement of chemiluminescence

The light yield from the chemiluminescent reaction can be measured using various parameters. These include peak light intensity (PLI); total light

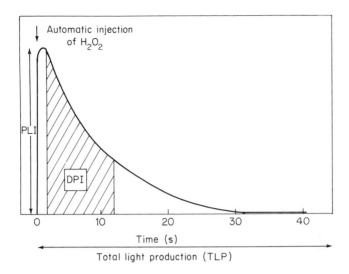

Fig. 5. Oscilloscope tracing of the light signal obtained upon oxidation of a chemiluminescent marker steroid conjugate with a H_2O_2 microperoxidase system at pH 13. PLI, peak light intensity; DPI, decay part integration

production (TLP) and decay part integration (DPI) (Fig. 5). The measurement of peak light intensity is simple. However, the kinetics of the chemiluminescence reaction are dependent upon the rapid and even mixing of the reagents which may modify the shape of the curve. Accordingly, to quantify chemiluminescence, it is preferable to integrate the peak area partially (Fig. 5, DPI), or completely (Fig. 5, TLP).

3.3. Advantages and disadvantages of chemiluminescent antigens

The most significant advantages of chemiluminescent tagged antigens are improved stability in comparison to radioactive tracers, safety, speed and sensitivity of detection, and a low cost per tube. On the other hand, the measurement of chemiluminescence is a more critical step than the measurement of radioactivity since the light signal generated by oxidation of the labelled antigen has to be initiated. Thus the sensitivity and precision of luminescence detection can be affected by several factors which include: (i) the presence of high background levels of luminescence in the reagents–consequently great care must be taken in the preparation of buffers; (ii) the quenching of light emission–the presence of materials of biological origin such as plasma or urine can modify the kinetics and cause scattering of the light emission (Tommasi et al., 1984), and (iii) the precision of injection–the volume of hydrogen peroxide and the speed of the injection in association with the size of the assay tube affect the rate of the chemiluminescence reaction. However, the use of a suitable luminometer equipped with an automatic dispenser (e.g. LKB Luminometer 1250 in conjunction with an automatic dispenser) or with an automated injection system (e.g. Lumac M2080) may avoid some of the problems associated with the injection of oxidant.

3.4. Variations of chemiluminescence immunoassay

We have used two main types of assay format: (i) systems that do not require physical separation of the antibody-bound and free analyte, i.e. homogenous or non-separation methods, and (ii) assays that require a separation step, i.e. heterogeneous or separation methods. Each type will be described separately.

3.4.1. Homogeneous chemiluminescence immunoassay

The basis of this assay is the finding that oxidation of the chemiluminescent marker conjugate in the presence of the homologous antibody (Kohen et al., 1979), or binding protein (Schroeder et al., 1976b) produces enhancement of chemiluminescence. In binding reactions the light enhancement is inhibited by homologous ligand in a dose-dependent manner (Kohen et al., 1979, 1982). Thus, this procedure obviates the need for separation of antibody-bound and free ligand. Assays based on this principle were developed for the measurement of progesterone (Kohen et al., 1979, 1981b) oestriol-16α-glucuronide (Kohen et al., 1980a), and oestriol (Kohen et al., 1981b). Although comparable sensitivity to RIA (5–10 pg per tube) was obtained, and the assay was amenable to automation, the homogeneous assay was affected by interference from luminescent compounds present in extracts of plasma or diluted urine. Moreover, in some systems the specific antibody did not enhance the light yield of the marker conjugate during oxidation. To overcome these problems, assays requiring the separation of bound and free ligand were developed.

3.4.2. Heterogeneous chemiluminescence immunoassay

In this type of assay the separation of antibody-bound and free fractions can be achieved either in the liquid or solid phase. The liquid phase includes the use of: (i) second antibody (Pratt et al., 1978); (ii) Sephadex G-25 columns (Schroeder et al., 1977), and (iii) more recently, Dextran-coated charcoal (Pazzagli et al., 1981b,c,d). The solid-phase methods include the use of immunoadsorption techniques and covalently coupled first or second antibodies. We shall consider systems using Dextran-coated charcoal for phase separation, and solid-phase techniques.

3.4.2.1. Use of Dextran-coated charcoal

This procedure can be applied to plasma or urinary extracts of steroids such as progesterone (Pazzagli *et al.*, 1981d), cortisol (Pazzagli *et al.*, 1981b) and testosterone (Pazzagli *et al.*, 1982) using the same antibody as the one used in a RIA system (Fig. 6). Sensitivity and precision similar to RIA were achieved. However, the assays may be affected by the presence of materials of biological origin (see Fig. 7). Moreover, Dextran-coated charcoal may cause stripping of the antibody-bound fraction. In order to overcome some of these problems, the use of an on-line computer analysis of the chemiluminescent reactions has been described (Tommasi *et al.*, 1984). In this system (see the block diagram in Fig. 8) the kinetics or shape of the chemiluminescent reaction is analysed for each measurement. Each chemiluminescent reaction is monitored, and samples that show quenching (e.g. reaction B or C in Fig. 7) are rejected in the final calculation of the results.

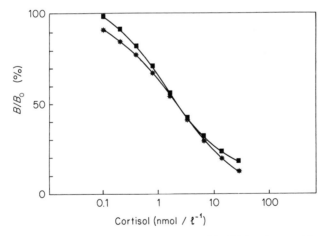

Fig. 6. Dose–response curves for cortisol as measured by RIA using a tritiated antigen or chemiluminescence immunoassay (CIA). The same antibody, and D extran-coated charcoal for phase separation were used. ■–■, CIA;★–★, RIA

3.4.2.2. Solid-phase methods

In these assays, the specific antibodies (monoclonal or polyclonal) are either adsorbed on the surface of polystyrene tubes or balls (Lindner *et al.*, 1981; Kohen *et al.*, 1982; Collins *et al.*, 1983), or covalently linked to polyacryla-

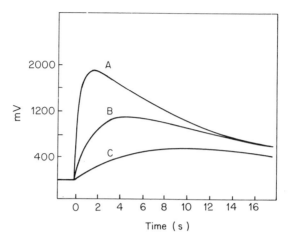

Fig. 7. Effect of urine on the light yield of cortisol-3-carboxymethyl oxime ethylisoluminol (100 fmol) obtained upon oxidation in the absence of urine (curve A) or in the presence of 10 μl (curve B) or 20 μl of urine (curve C)

mide beads (Kohen and Lindner, 1983; Kohen *et al.*, 1983). In the immunoadsorption method, aspiration of the reaction mixture and subsequent washing with buffer removed all potentially interfering substances with the concomitant reduction of background chemiluminescence. This approach is simple and has enabled the development of assays for the measurement of

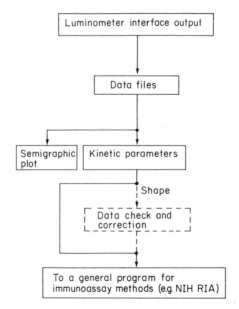

Fig. 8. Block diagram of the microcomputer–luminometer system

urinary steroid metabolites such a pregnanediol-3α-glucuronide (Eshhar *et al.*, 1981; Barnard *et al.*, 1981b), oestriol-16α-glucuronide (Barnard *et al.*, 1981a), oestrone-3-glucuronide (Weerasekera *et al.*, 1982) and plasma steroids such as progesterone (Kohen *et al.*, 1981a), oestradiol (Kim *et al.*, 1982) and testosterone (Collins *et al.*, 1983).

Although this technique can be considered a single tube assay, it has certain disadvantages such as: (i) the method is antibody consumptive and has slower kinetics; (ii) the amount of antibody that can be attached to a tube is subject to a physical limit; (iii) some antibodies once coated on a plastic surface fail to retain their immunoreactivity; (iv) the support may show a batch to batch variation, and (v) the antibody-coated tubes may lose stability upon storage. On the other hand, the use of antibodies covalently coupled to polyacrylamide beads eliminated some of the problems associated with the immunoadsorption techniques. The advantages of this methods are as follows: (i) the antibodies retain their immunoreactivity after conjugation and are stable in solution at 4 °C or in a lyophilized form; (ii) the reaction rates are fast, and (iii) it is possible to maintain good precision and quality control.

Subsequently, we developed solid-phase assays incorporating the following features (Kohen *et al.*, 1983): (i) a steroid–chemiluminescent marker conjugate as the labelled ligand; (ii) polyclonal or monoclonal antibodies covalently coupled to polymer beads as the specific immunoadsorbent, and (iii) a centrifugation step after the binding reaction to remove interfering luminescent compounds together with unbound steroid. The chemiluminescent reaction (oxidation of the bound fraction with H_2O_2 and microperoxidase) is performed at pH 13 under conditions that maximize the quantum yield. A simplified flow diagram of the method is shown in Fig. 9. Representative examples will be given below for plasma steroids and urinary steroid metabolites.

3.4.2.2.1 Plasma steroids

Chemiluminescence-based immunoassays were developed for the measurement of plasma testosterone (Kohen *et al.*, 1983) and plasma oestradiol (De Boever *et al.*, 1983) using the method summarized in Fig. 9. The labelled antigens were testosterone-3-[O]-carboxymethyl oxime aminobutylethylisoluminol and oestradiol-6-[O]-carboxymethyl oxime aminobutylethylisoluminol respectively. The immunoadsorbent in each case consisted of monoclonal antibodies to the homologous hapten coupled covalently to polyacrylamide beads. Sensitive dose–response curves for both steroids were obtained and an example for oestradiol is given in Fig. 10.

The assay results conformed closely with those obtained by a RIA for oestradiol ($r = 0.94$; $n = 105$), and for testosterone ($r = 0.98$; $n = 35$). The oestradiol assay was used to monitor ovulation induction during gonadotrophin therapy (De Boever *et al.*, 1983). The precision of the solid-phase

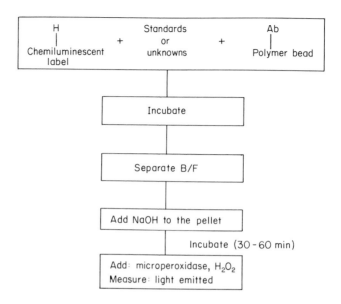

Fig. 9. A flow diagram of the solid-phase chemiluminescence immunoassay method.
H, hormone; B, bound; F, free

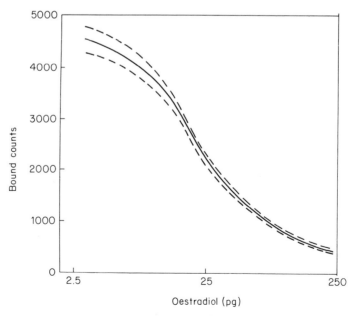

Fig. 10. A dose–response curve for oestradiol as measured by chemiluminescence
immunoassay, ———, mean counts; ---, error envelope, i.e. ± 2 S.D.

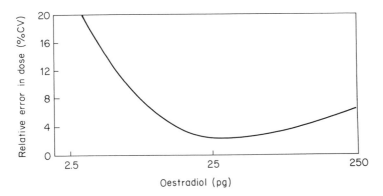

Fig. 11. Precision profile for the oestradiol chemiluminescence immunoassay corrected for use of duplicates

chemiluminescence immunoassay for plasma oestradiol (the intra-assay and the inter-assay coefficients of variation were less than 10%) and the limits of detection (5 pg per tube) were comparable to those of RIA. The precision profile of the chemiluminescence immunoassay for plasma oestradiol was similar to that of RIA (Fig. 11).

3.4.2.2.2. Urinary steroid metabolites

We have developed direct, solid-phase chemiluminescence immunoassays for two urinary steroid metabolites for monitoring ovarian function in women. These are oestra-1,3,5(10)-triene-17-one-3α-D-glucopyranosiduronic acid (oestrone-3-glucuronide; E_1-3G) (Kohen et al., 1983) and 5β-pregnane-3α,20α-diol-3α-D-glucopyranosiduronic acid (pregnanediol-3α-glucuronide; Pd-3α-G) (Kohen et al., 1983). The labelled antigens were E_1-3-G aminoethylisoluminol and Pd-3α-G aminohexylethylisoluminol. The E_1-3-G assay was developed by using polyclonal rabbit anti-E_1-3-G antibodies conjugated to the immunobead matrix; whereas the Pd-3α-G assay was developed using the second antibody (goat anti-mouse IgG) conjugated to polymer beads.

Using these assays, the pre-ovulatory rise of E_1-3-G (Fig. 12) and the post-ovulatory rise of Pd-3α-G during the normal human menstrual cycle were determined (Kohen et al., 1983). These methods provide a simple, non-invasive approach to monitor ovarian function. Moreover, recent findings indicate that the measurement of E_1-3-G may be a reliable biochemical index for the determination of the start and finish of the fertile period (Weerasekera et al., 1982). Furthermore, the oestrogenic response of amenorrhoeic patients to treatment with human postmenopausal urine gonadotropin can be conveniently monitored by measurement of E_1-3-G concentra-

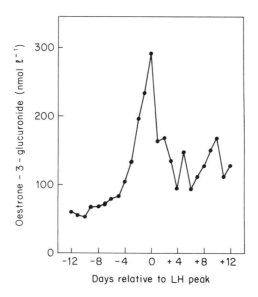

Fig. 12. Mean daily excretion of oestrone-3-glucuronide in samples of eary morning urine throughout 10 normal menstrual cycles as determined by chemiluminescence immunoassay

tions in early morning samples of urine (Kohen *et al.*, 1983). The precision, specificity and reproducibility of the chemiluminescence immunoassay for E_1-3-G and for Pd-3α-G were comparable to those of RIA (Kohen *et al.*, 1983).

4.   BIOLUMINESCENCE IMMUNOASSAY

In this type of assay bioluminescent labels such as bacterial or firefly luciferase have been used for labelling antigens (Wannlund *et al.*, 1980; Wannlund and DeLuca, 1981). Alternatively, co-factors ATP or NAD that will participate directly in a bioluminescent reaction have been used for tagging antigens (Carrico *et al.*, 1976a,b, 1978). Schematic outlines of firefly and bacterial luminescence reactions are shown in Figs. 13 and 14 respectively.

$$\text{ligand–ATP} + O_2 + \text{Luciferin}$$
$$|$$
$$\text{Luciferase}$$
$$\downarrow$$
$$\text{Oxyluciferin} + \text{AMP} + CO_2 + \text{PPi} + \text{Green Light (562 nm)}$$

Fig. 13. Reaction sequence of the firefly bioluminescence system using co-factor-labelled haptens

(i) Substrate + Ligand–NAD $\xrightarrow{\text{dehydrogenase}}$ Ligand–NADH + Products

(ii) Ligand–NADH $\xrightarrow{\text{NADH:FMN oxidoreductase}}$ Ligand–NAD + $FMNH_2$

(iii) $FMNH_2$ + O_2 + Long-chain aldehyde $\xrightarrow{\text{Luciferase}}$ FMN + RCO_2H + Blue light
                                                                    (495 nm)

Fig. 14. Bacterial bioluminescence using co-factor labelled haptens

The availability of highly purified bioluminescence reagents is a prerequisite for the development of immunoassays utilizing these systems. Nevertheless, bioluminescence immunoassays have certain advantages which include: (i) the achievement of a high quantum yield and (ii) the stable emission
of light. The second feature avoids the necessity for an automatic injection
system. For these reasons we attempted to devise bioluminescent immunoassays for steroids utilizing NAD-labelled haptens. A brief description of this
approach is given below.

4.1. Synthesis of Co-factor Labelled Steroids

Carboxy derivatives of steroids or urinary steroid glucuronides were conjugated to an aminoethyl derivative of nicotinamide adenine dinucleotide
(AE-NAD) in a two-step procedure (Kohen et al., 1978) via an activated
steroid ester derivative. The resulting marker conjugates were purified by
high voltage electrophoresis. The coenzymatic activity of these conjugates
was determined using the reactions depicted in Fig. 14. In comparison to
unaltered NAD^+, these conjugates retained 5–10% of the activity. In
addition the binding affinity of the labelled antigens towards the homologous
antibody ranged from 40–60%.

4.2. Bioluminescence Immunoassay for Oestriol-16α-glucuronide

A homogeneous bioluminescence immunoassay for oestriol-16α-glucuronide
was developed (Barnard, 1982), using the labelled conjugate shown in Fig. 15
and the flow diagram depicted in Fig. 16. The basis of this assay is the finding
that bioluminescence from the bacterial luciferase system is significantly
reduced when the hapten–cofactor conjugate is bound to the homologous
antibody. In competitive binding reactions the inhibition of the light yield is
reversed by the presence of homologous hapten in a dose-dependent manner.
The assay, performed in the liquid phase, is simple and does not require the
separation of the antibody-bound and free forms of the analyte. A typical
dose–response curve for oestriol-16α-glucuronide is shown in Fig. 17. This
assay, at present, is unsuitable for the measurement of oestriol-16α-

O
C—N—CH2
H
OH
O
O
HO
OH
CH2
HO
O
NH
C-NH2
N
N
N
N
N
R—P—P—R

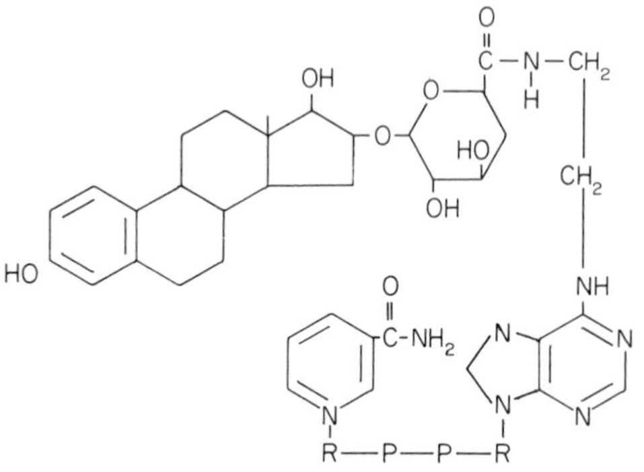

Fig. 15. Proposed structure for oestriol-16α-glucuronide aminoethyl NAD conjugate. R, ribose; P, phosphate

glucuronide in diluted urine because other components inhibit the activity of the bioluminescent reagents, and the sensitivity of the assay is one order of magnitude less than a heterogeneous chemiluminescence immunoassay.

The incorporation of a separation step into the bioluminescence immunoassay, followed by the addition of authentic analyte to displace the labelled antigen from the antibodies, improves the assay performance (Barnard, 1982). More recently, Hughes *et al.* (1984) have described the synthesis of progesterone-3-carboxymethyl oxime–NAD for use in a homogeneous assay

1. Pre-reduce label
E3-16α-G-AENAD
Glucose-6-phosphate
6-Phosphogluconate
Glucose 6-phosphate dehydrogenase (Sigma type 24)
E3-16α-G-AENADH
2. Pre-incubate
Antibody + Standard/sample, 10 mins
3. Add labelled antigen (2ng)
Incubate 10 min
4. Add bioluminescence monitoring reagent
(Luciferase/FMN/C10 aldehyde); mix
5. Integrate signal

Fig. 16. A schematic diagram of the homogeneous bioluminescence immunoassay for oestriol-16α-glucuronide

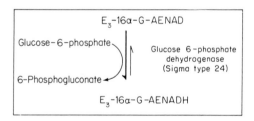

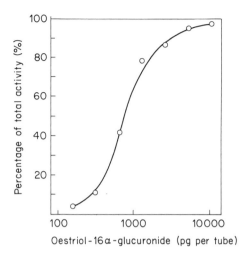

Fig. 17. A dose–response curve for oestriol-16α-glucuronide as measured by bioluminescence immunoassay

based on antibody-enhanced bioluminescence for the measurement of plasma progesterone. Currently, we are investigating the use of biotin as an indirect probe for haptens, with biotinylated glucose 6-phosphate dehydrogenase as the labelled reagent. Streptavidin is used to link the biotinylated hapten to the biotinylated enzyme. In the presence of substrate (i.e. glucose 6-phosphate) the enzyme converts NAD to $NADH_2$, which may be monitored according to the reactions shown in Fig. 14 (Kohen et al., 1984).

5. CONCLUDING REMARKS

The work reviewed here indicates that it is feasible to use chemiluminescence-based immunoassays for the determination of steroids and their metabolites in biological fluids. The procedures are comparable to established RIA in terms of sensitivity, specificity, accuracy and precision. However, the setting up of the present technology in the routine clinical laboratory is more complex than the establishment of RIA procedures. This limitation is due to several components of the assay, such as the structure and the affinity of the labelled antigen, the type of antibody and the technique used for phase separation. For example, the length of the spacer between the steroid and the isoluminol plays a role in the light yield obtained upon oxidation of the marker conjugate. In the case of conjugates of oestrone-3-glucuronide (Weerasekera et al., 1982) and progesterone, a short chain of two methylene groups between the steroid and isoluminol was found to be preferable to a larger chain of four or six methylene groups. In certain instances, the marker conjugate (e.g. progesterone-11α-hemisuccinyl ABEI conjugate), shows a higher affinity towards the homologous antibody than tritiated progesterone (Pazzagli *et al.*, 1981c). Thus, proper selection of the marker conjugate is an absolute necessity. Furthermore, it is also important to match the antibody used (monoclonal or polyclonal) with the particular marker conjugate. Differences in sensitivity have been observed between polyclonal and monoclonal antibodies. For instance, the use of specific monoclonal antibodies to testosterone (Kohen *et al.*, 1983) in the assay yielded a very sensitive dose–response curve. In addition, the use of monoclonal antibodies in non-isotopic immunoassays for haptens ensures that the labelled antigen and analyte compete for the same binding sites.

Another factor to be considered is the technique used for the separation of antibody-bound and free forms of labelled antigen. When charcoal is used for phase separation, the possible luminescent interfering substances remaining in the soluble bound fraction have to be considered. In this case, an on-line computer may identify some of the problems (Tommasi *et al.*, 1984). The interference from luminescent compounds present in plasma extracts or diluted urine can be overcome by the use of solid phase techniques.

Another limitation of assays using isoluminol derivatives is the final oxidation of the label at high pH (see last step in Fig. 9). Sodium hydroxide is added to the antibody-bound label for the following reasons: (i) to raise the pH so that the light yield is enhanced and the sensitivity of the assay is improved, and (ii) to dissociate the antibody-bound complex. The enhancement of chemiluminescence necessitates an extra incubation step (see Fig. 9). Each assay has to be optimized with respect to the concentration of sodium hydroxide together with the time and incubation temperature of the reaction.

Despite these limitations, chemiluminescence-based immunoassays do provide a viable alternative to radioimmunoassays and the methods avoid the use of a radioactive label. Future developments in this area will include: (i) alternative probes that may lead to constant, stable light emissions; (ii) simpler oxidation systems for derivatives of isoluminol, and (iii) alternative chemiluminescence labels such as acridinium ester derivatives (Weeks *et al.*, 1983a,b). Additional applications of chemiluminescence immunoassays for haptens, and the development of immunochemiluminometric assays for proteins are described in Chapters 3, 9 and 10 in this volume.

ACKNOWLEDGEMENTS

We are grateful to Drs G. Barnard, J. B. Kim, W. P. Collins, G. Messeri, A. Tommasi, M. Damiani and Z. Eshhar for permission to quote collaborative work; to Mrs S. Lichter, Mrs B. Gaier, Mrs J. Ausher, Mr A. Almoznino, Mrs S. Gilad and Mrs D. Leyseale for technical assistance; to Mrs M. Kopelowitz for excellent secretarial assistance; to the special Programme of

Research, Development and Research Training, World Health Organization, the Bosch Foundation and the Rockefeller Foundation for financial support, and to Drs W. Coulson and P. Samarajeewa, the Courtauld Institute of Biochemistry, The Middlesex Hospital Medical School, London, for the steroid glucuronides used in this study.

REFERENCES

Barnard, G., Collins, W. P., Kohen, F. and Lindner, H. R. (1981a). The measurement of urinary estriol-16α-glucuronide by a solid-phase chemiluminescence immunoassay. *J. Steroid Biochem.* **14**, 941–948.

Barnard, G., Collins, W. P., Kohen, F. and Lindner, H. R. (1981b). A preliminary study of the measurement of urinary pregnanediol-3α-glucuronide by a solid-phase chemiluminescence immunoassay. In *Bioluminescence and Chemiluminescence* (W. D. McElroy and M. A. DeLuca, eds), Academic Press, New York, pp. 311–317.

Barnard, G. J. (1982). Technological developments in immunoassay. PhD thesis, University of London.

Carrico, R. J., Christner, J. E., Boguslaski, R. C. and Yeung, K. K. (1976a). A method for monitoring specific binding reactions with cofactor labelled ligands. *Analyt. Biochem.*, **72**, 271–282.

Carrico, R. J., Yeung, K. K., Schroeder, H. R., Boguslaski, R. C., Buckler, R. T. and Christner, J. E. (1976b). Specific protein-binding reactions monitored with ligand–ATP conjugates and firefly luciferase. *Analyt. Biochem.*, **76**, 95–110.

Carrico, R. J., Johnson, R. D. and Boguslaski, R. C. (1978). ATP-labelled ligands and firefly luciferase for monitoring specific protein-binding reactions. *Meth. Enzymol.*, **57**, 113–133.

Collins, W. P., Barnard, G. J., Kim, J. B., Weerasekera, D. A., Kohen, F., Eshhar, Z. and Lindner, H. R. (1983). Chemiluminescence immunoassays for plasma steroids and urinary steroid metabolites. In *Immunoassays for Clinical Chemistry: A Workshop Meeting, Edinburgh, March 1982* (W. M. Hunter and J. E. T. Corrie, eds), Churchill Livingstone, Edinburgh, pp. 373–397.

De Boever, J., Kohen, F. and Vanderkerckhove, D. (1983). A solid phase chemiluminescence immunoassay for plasma estradiol-17β for gonadotropin therapy compared with two different radioimmunoassays. *Clin. Chem.* **29**, 2068–2072.

Eshhar, Z., Kim, J. B., Barnard, G., Collins, W. P., Gilad, S., Lindner, H.R. and Kohen, F. (1981). Use of monoclonal antibodies to pregnanediol-3α-glucuronide for the development of a solid-phase chemiluminescence immunoassay. *Steroids*, **38**, 89–106.

Hughes, J., Short, F. and James, V. H. T. (1984). Synthesis of a novel bioluminescent conjugate of progesterone for immunoassay. In *Analytical Applications of Bioluminescence and Chemiluminescence* (L. Kricka, P. E. Stanley, G. H. G. Thorpe and T. Whitehead, eds), Academic Press, New York, pp. 269–272.

Kim, J. B., Barnard, G. J., Collins, W. P., Kohen, F., Lindner, H. R. and Eshhar, Z. (1982). Measurement of plasma estradiol-17β by solid-phase chemiluminescence immunoassay. *Clin. Chem.*, **28**, 1120–1124.

Kohen, F. and Lindner, H. R. (1983). Metodi immunoluminescenti in fase solida. In *Luminsecenza* (M. Pazzagli, ed.), OIC Medical Press, Firenze, pp. 83–100.

Kohen, F., Hollander, Z., Yeager, F. M., Carrico, R. J. and Boguslaski, R. C. (1978). A homogeneous enzyme immunoassay for estriol monitored by coenzymic cycling reactions. In *Enzyme Labelled Immunoassay of Hormones and Drugs* (S. B. Pal, ed.), Walter de Gruyter, Berlin, pp. 69–75.

Kohen, F., Passagli, M., Kim, J. B., Lindner, H. R. and Boguslaski, R. C. (1979). An assay procedure for plasma progesterone based on antibody enhanced chemiluminescence. *FEBS Lett.*, **104**, 201–205.

Kohen, F., Kim, J. B., Barnard, G. and Lindner, H. R. (1980a). An immunoassay for urinary estriol-16α-glucuronide based on antibody-enhanced chemiluminescence. *Steroids*, **36**, 405–419.

Kohen, F., Pazzagli, M., Kim, J. B. and Lindner, H. R. (1980b). An immunoassay for plasma cortisol based on chemiluminescence. *Steroids*, **36**, 421–438.

Kohen, F., Kim, J. B., Lindner, H. R. and Collins, W. P. (1981a). Development of a solid-phase chemiluminescence immunoassay for plasma progesterone. *Steroids*, **38**, 73–88.

Kohen, F., Kim, J. B. and Lindner, H. R. (1981b). Assay of gonadal steroids based on antibody-enhanced chemiluminescence. In *Bioluminescence and Chemiluminescence* (W. D. McElroy and M. A. DeLuca, eds), Academic Press, New York, pp. 357–364.

Kohen, F., Kim, J. B., Lindner, H. R. and Eshhar, Z. (1982). Steroid immunoassays using chemiluminescent labels. In *Luminescent Assays: Perspectives in Endocrinology and Clinical Chemistry* (M. Serio and M. Pazzagli, eds), Raven Press, New York, pp. 169–179.

Kohen, F., Lindner, H. R. and Gilad, S. (1983). Development of chemiluminescence monitored immunoassays for steroid hormones. *J. Steroid Biochem.*, **19**, 413–418.

Kohen, F., Bayer, E. A., Wilchek, M., Barnard, G., Kim, J. B., Collins, W. P., Beheshti, I., Richardson, A. and McCapra, F. (1984). Development of luminescence-based immunoassays for haptens and for peptide hormones. In *Analytical Applications of Bioluminescence and Chemiluminescence* (L. Kricka, P. E. Stanley, G. H. G. Thorpe and T. P. Whitehead, eds). Academic Press, New York, pp. 149–158.

Kricka, J. L. and Carter, T. J. N. (1982). Luminescent immunoassays. In *Clinical and Biochemical Luminescence* (L. J. Kricka and T. J. N. Carter, eds), Marcel Dekker, New York, pp. 153–178.

Lindner, H. R., Kohen, F., Eshhar, Z., Kim, J. B., Barnard, G. and Collins, W. P. (1981). Novel assay procedure for assessing ovarian function in women. *J. Steroid Biochem.* **15**, 131–136.

Maier, C. (1977). Luminescent conjugates for immunological analysis: comprising a complex formed between a pharmacologically, immunologically or biochemically active ligand and a chemiluminescent compound. Belgian Patent no. 856,182.

Maier, C. L. (1978). Procedure for the assay of pharmacologically, immunologically and biochemically active compounds in biological fluids. US Patent no. 4,104,029.

Pazzagli, M., Kim, J. B., Messeri, G., Kohen, F., Bolelli, G. F., Tommasi, A., Salerno, R., Monetti, G. and Serio, M. (1981a). Luminescence immunoassay (LIA) or cortisol. 1. Synthesis and evaluation of the chemiluminescent labels of cortisol. *J. Steroid Biochem.* **14**, 1005–1012.

Pazzagli, M., Kim, J. B., Messeri, G., Kohen, F., Bolelli, G. F., Tommasi, A., Salerno, R. and Serio, M. (1981b). Luminescent immunoassay (LIA) or cortisol. 2. Development and validation of the immunoassay monitored by chemiluminescence. *J. Steroid Biochem.* **14**, 1181–1187.

Pazzagli, M., Kim, J. B., Messeri, G., Martinazzo, G., Kohen, F., Francheschetti, F., Monetti, G., Salerno, R. Tommasi, A. and Serio, M. (1981c). Evaluation of different progesterone–isoluminol conjugates for chemiluminescence immunoassay. *Clin. Chim. Acta* **115**, 277–286.

Pazzagli, M., Kim, J. B., Messeri, G., Martinazzo, G., Kohen, F., Francheschetti, F., Tommasi, A., Salerno, R. and Serio, M. (1981d). Luminescent immunoassay (LIA) for progesterone in a heterogeneous system. *Clin. chim. Acta*, **115**, 287–296.

Pazzagli, M., Serio, M., Munsun, P. and Rodbard, D. (1982). A chemiluminescent immunoassay (LIA) for testosterone. In *Radioimmunoassay and Related Procedures in Medicine*, IAEA, Vienna, pp. 747–755.

Pazzagli, M., Messeri, G., Caldini, A. L., Monetic, G., Martinazzo, G. and Serio, M. (1983). Preparation and evaluation of steroid chemiluminescent tracers. *J. Steroid Biochem*. **19**, 407–412.

Pratt, J. J., Woldring, M. G. and Villerius, L. (1978). Chemiluminescence-linked immunoassay. *J. Immunol. Meth*. **21**, 179–184.

Schroeder, H. R. and Yeager, F. M. (1978). Chemiluminescence yields and detection limits of some iso-luminol derivatives in various oxidation systems. *Analyt. Chem*. **50**, 1114–1120.

Schroeder, H. R., Carrico, R. J., Boguslaski, R. C. and Christner, J. E. (1976a). Specific binding reactions monitored with ligand–cofactor conjugates and bacterial luciferase. *Analyt. Biochem*. **72**, 283–292.

Schroeder, H. R., Vogelhut, P. O., Carrico, R. J., Boguslaski, R. C. and Buckler, R. T. (1976b). Competitive protein binding assay for biotin monitored by chemiluminescence. *Analyt. Chem*. **48**, 1933–1937.

Schroeder, H. R., Yeager, F. M., Boguslaski, R. C., Snoke, E. O. and Buckler, R. T. (1977). Immunoassay for thyroxine monitored by chemiluminescence. *Clin. Chem*. **23**, 1132–1136.

Schroeder, H. R., Boguslaski, R. C., Carrico, R. J. and Buckler, R. T. (1978). Monitoring specific protein-binding reactions with chemiluminescence. *Meth. Enzymol*. **57**, 424–445.

Schroeder, H. R., Yeager, F. M., Boguslaski, R. C. and Vogelhut, P. O. (1979). Immunoassay for serum thyroxine monitored by chemiluminescence. *J. Immunol. Meth*. **25**, 275–282.

Tommasi, A., Pazzagli, M., Damiani, M., Salerno, R., Messeri, G, Magini, A. and Serio, M. (1984). On-line computer analyses of chemiluminescent reactions with applications to a luminescent immunoassay for free cortisol in urine. *Clin. Chem*. **30**, 1597–1602.

Wannlund, J., Azari, J., Levine, L. and DeLuca, M. (1980). A bioluminescent immunoassay for methotrexate at the subpicomole level. *Biochem. Biophys. Res. Commun*. **96**, 440–446.

Wannlund, J. and DeLuca, M. (1981). Bioluminescent immunoassays: use of luciferase-antigen conjugates for determination of methotrexate and DNP. In *Bioluminescence and Chemiluminescence* (M. A. DeLuca and W. D. McElroy, eds), Academic Press, New York, pp. 693–696.

Weeks, I., Beheshti, I., McCapra, F., Campbell, A. K. and Woodhead, J. S. (1983a). Acridinium esters as high-specific-activity labels in immunoassay. *Clin. Chem*. **29**, 1474–1479.

Weeks, I., Campbell, A. K. and Woodhead, J. S. (1983b). Two-site immunochemiluminometric assay for human α-fetoprotein. *Clin. Chem*. **29**, 1480–1483.

Weerasekera, D. A., Kim, J. B., Barnard, G., J., Collins, W. P., Kohen, F. and Lindner, H. R. (1982). Monitoring ovarian function by a solid-phase chemiluminescence immunoassay. *Acta Endocr. Copenh*. **101**, 254–263.

Whitehead, T. P., Thorpe, G. H. G., Carter, T. J. N., Groucutt, C., and Kricka, L. J. (1983). Enhanced luminescence procedure for sensitive determination of peroxidase-labelled conjugates in immunoassay. *Nature, Lond*. **305**, 158–159.

Alternative Immunoassays
Edited by W. P. Collins
© 1985 John Wiley & Sons Ltd

CHAPTER 9

Chemiluminescence immunoassays and immunochemiluminometric assays

G. J. R. Barnard, J. B. Kim and J. L. Williams

*Department of Obstetrics and Gynaecology,
Diagnostics Research Unit,
King's College School of Medicine and Dentistry,
Denmark Hill, London SE5 8RX, UK*

1. INTRODUCTION

The principal aims of this chapter are to describe various chemiluminescence immunoassays (CIAs) in detail and to discuss current and future developments of the technique which include alternative approaches to the measurement of haptens in a variety of body fluids and the development of direct (non-extraction) assays. In addition, descriptions are given of several methods for the measurement of protein hormones in plasma or urine, which involve CIA or immunochemiluminometric assay (ICMA).

1.1. Established procedures

In 1976, Schroeder *et al.* described a competitive protein binding assay for biotin which was monitored by chemiluminescence. It was found that the light emitted from the oxidation of biotinyl-isoluminol was enhanced upon binding to avidin and the signal was decreased in the presence of increasing amounts of authentic biotin. More recently, homogeneous or non-separation immunoassays have been reported for the measurement of plasma steroids and their urinary metabolites after a preliminary purification of the sample (Kohen *et al.*, 1979, 1980a,b). Homogeneous assays have several advantages which include: (i) simplicity; (ii) speed; (iii) the potential to be more precise, and (iv) ease of automation. The fundamental problem associated with this type of assay, however, is the interference with the end-point determination by components of the biological samples.

A heterogeneous (or separation) CIA, which eliminated the effect of interfering compounds in the biological sample was developed by Barnard *et al.* (1981) for the measurement of pregnanediol-3α-glucuronide in diluted urine. Since that time, several solid-phase and liquid-phase separation CIAs for the measurement of haptens have been developed and evaluated (see Chapter 8 in this volume).

1.2. The measurement of chemiluminescence

The light output from a chemiluminescent reagent may be measured simply with high sensitivity (see Chapter 7 in this volume).

1.2.1. Apparatus

The essential components for the measurement and recording of chemiluminescence are shown in Fig. 1. The sample chamber must be designed to collect the maximum amount of light from the reaction mixture. Extraneous sources of light are excluded and the housing is maintained at constant temperature. The sample must be rapidly and reproducibly mixed with the reagent which initiates the chemiluminescence, and the photomultiplier tube and mirror must be placed in the optimum position relative to the reaction vessel. An amplifier is required to drive the output devices, which may include both analogue and digital displays. The construction of different instruments for the measurement of chemiluminescence and bioluminescence has been reviewed (Anderson *et al.*, 1978).

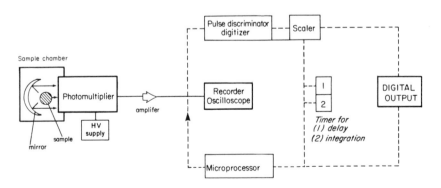

Fig. 1. Essential features of chemiluminescence monitoring equipment

1.2.2. Factors affecting the measurement of chemiluminescence

The sensitivity and precision of luminescence detection is affected by several factors:

(i) *The presence of high background luminescence* Great care must be taken in the selection of pure reagents since small amounts of impurity may give high background luminescence which greatly reduces the sensitivity of detection. In particular, the purity of the water used in the preparation of buffers is critical. It is our experience that deionized water should be avoided and that double distillation in glass produces the best results. In addition, it is recommended that chemical syntheses involving milligram quantities of luminescent material should be performed in laboratory space that is physically separated from the area where immunoassay procedures are carried out.

(ii) *The quenching of light emission* The types of buffers and their constituents, in particular bovine serum albumin and sodium azide, markedly affect the degree to which the chemiluminescence reaction is quenched. The sample itself may also change the spectral distribution of the emission, particularly if it is highly coloured or contains fluorescent compounds. This problem is more apparent in homogeneous assays. In addition, the presence of particles in a biological sample may cause the light to be scattered and lost.

(iii) *The precision of injection* The volume of oxidant and the injection rate in association with assay tube size affect the reaction kinetics. This effect is minimized if the light signal is integrated. If the method is dependent on peak height analysis, however, good precision of repeated injections is essential. Certain commercial luminescence photometers are committed to the use of very narrow glass tubes which may be unsuitable for the chemiluminescence reaction.

(iv) *The efficiency of photodetection* This facet depends on the geometry and state of the sample housing, the photomultiplier tube and the associated electronic circuits. The most sensitive photomultipliers have a cathode efficiency of approximately 20%. The speed of response and the wavelength of the emitted light will affect the efficiency of detection which can be obtained from any particular instrument using a standard light source (Seliger, 1978). Stabilizer circuits may be necessary to reduce the effect of changes in power supply.

1.2.3. Instruments used in chemiluminescence immunoassay

Several luminescence photometers are available commercially. The ideal instrument for solid-phase and liquid-phase CIAs should have the following features: (i) the facility to receive a wide variety of tubes or cuvettes; (ii) the automatic injection of at least one reagent (e.g. hydrogen peroxide); (iii) the availability of flexible integration; (iv) a digital display and/or printout; (v) an optional flat-bed recorder; (vi) high sensitivity with good stability; (vii) a relatively low cost, and (viii) easy maintenance.

The instrument that we have used in the development, evaluation and routine adoption of CIA is the LKB Luminometer Model 1250 (see Fig. 2) and display (kindly provided by LKB Wallac, Turku, Finland), electronically linked to an automatic dispenser (Fig. 3; Hook and Tucker Instruments Ltd, Croydon, Surrey, UK). Care should be taken that the plastic reagent tubing which leads from the dispenser to the luminometer is protected from the light by a covering of black sleeving or aluminium foil and that clean white reflecting paper is correctly positioned in the cuvette holder. If necessary the holder may be fitted with an adapter to accommodate different assay tubes. In addition the internal standard can be set using the gain control and the value recorded for each assay. The light signal is measured over 10 s.

2. THE MEASUREMENT OF HAPTENS USING ISOLUMINOL DERIVATIVES

2.1. Liquid-phase, heterogeneous assays

Recently, we adopted the use of Dextran-coated charcoal for the separation step in CIAs for the routine measurement of various haptens in extracts of peripheral venous plasma and in diluted urine (Kim, 1983). After the

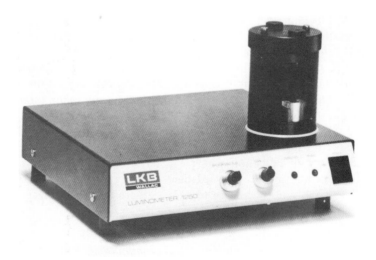

Fig. 2. The LKB Luminometer 1250

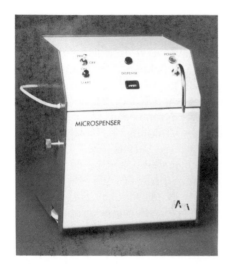

Fig. 3. The Hook and Tucker Microspenser

antibody-binding reaction (300 µl incubation volume), 200 µl of Dextran-coated charcoal (500 mg Norit A charcoal and 50 mg Dextran T 70 in 100 ml of assay buffer) are added, the contents mixed on a vortex mixer and incubated for 10 min at room temperature. The tubes are centrifuged (10 min; 2000g) and 200 µl of each supernatant are transferred to luminometer cuvettes containing 100 µl of 2 M sodium hydroxide. After incubation at 60 °C for 60 min, the cuvettes are cooled to room temperature. Microperoxidase solution (100 µl; 20 µg ml^{-1}) is added to each cuvette, which is immediately placed in the luminometer, and chemiluminescence is initiated by the injection of 100 µl of 0.3% hydrogen peroxide. Long-term quality control data have been accumulated for the routine measurement of oestradiol, progesterone and testosterone in extracts of peripheral plasma by CIA and these are shown in Table 1.

Table 1. Routine CIA of steroids: long-term quality control

	No. of batches	QC1 †			QC2 †		
		Mean	s.d.	CV (%)	Mean	s.d.	CV (%)
Oestradiol (pmol 1^{-1})	16	111	16	14.4	1 826	165	9.0
Testosterone (nmol 1^{-1})	10	2.3	0.3	13.0	11.8	1.2	10.2
Progesterone (nmol 1^{-1})	30	10.8	1.9	17.6	16.7	1.0	6.0

† QCI and QC2 are pools of plasma for quality control

2.2. Solid-phase, heterogeneous assays

A variety of supports have been used in solid-phase CIA and include: (i) polystyrene tubes (LP 3; Luckham Ltd, Labro Works, Victoria Gardens, Burgess Hill, Sussex, UK); (ii) polypropylene tubes (catalogue no. 55.535; Sarstedt (UK) Ltd. 68 Boston Road, Beaumont Leys, Leicester, UK); and (iii) nylon and etched polystyrene beads (Northumbria Biologicals Ltd, South Nelson Industrial Estate, Cramlington, Northumberland, UK). Polystyrene beads have a relatively large surface area and efficiently adsorb the IgG fraction. In addition, the coated beads are easy to prepare and store.

Recently, methods have been devised which involve the use of second antibody coated tubes or beads (donkey anti-rabbit or goat anti-mouse) to provide an activated surface that can be prepared in sufficient quantities to meet the requirements of several different assays (Brockelbank et al., 1984). The advantages of this approach are: (i) the second antibody is coated in excess leading to improved precision, and (ii) the second antibody-binding reaction proceeds at the same time as the first avoiding prolonged incubation times.

To prepare the coated tubes, 200 μl of the IgG fraction (suitably diluted in barbital buffer) are added to each tube. Alternatively, polystyrene beads are added to the diluted IgG in the ratio one bead : 200 μl buffer. After an overnight incubation at 4 °C, the buffer is aspirated to waste and 0.3% BSA in saline added (200 μl per bead or tube). After an incubation of 30 min at room temperature (22 °C) the solution is aspirated to waste. The tubes are stored at 4 °C until required; the beads are stored in assay buffer at 4 °C. The beads are conveniently transferred from the bottle to the assay tube by means of a Pasteur pipette connected to a vacuum line. Treatment of the solid phase with 0.3% BSA in saline reduces the non-specific binding of labelled antigen and increases the stability of the coated antibody upon storage. Tubes and beads prepared in this way retain their activity for at least one year if stored at 4 °C.

One of the arguments against the use of antisera passively adsorbed to plastic surfaces has been the batch to batch variation in the manufacture of the raw materials. For example, in the case of polystyrene tubes obtained from one supplier at least three types have been identified by the colour of the tube. It has been demonstrated that any particular antibody will behave differently depending on the type of tube used. Consequently, it has been necessary to determine the preferred plastic for each assay. Particulate solid phases covalently linked to second antibodies have been used in a variety of CIAs to obviate the disadvantages of using plastic surfaces and the passive adsorption of specific IgG. The reagents which have been used include sheep anti-rabbit IgG attached to polyacrylamide beads (Immunobeads; Bio-Rad Laboratories Ltd, Watford, Herts, UK), or to small uniform plastic microspheres (Amerlex; Amersham International, Amersham, Berks, UK) and donkey anti-mouse IgG attached to fine particles of cellulose (Sac-cel; Wellcome Diagnostics Ltd, Dartford, Kent, UK).

A variety of solid phases have been used for the measurement of steroids in extracts of peripheral venous plasma, and the direct assay of analytes in saliva and serum.

2.3. Plasma oestradiol – extraction assay, antibody-coated tube separation

The oestradiol assay has been selected as a model for the evaluation of CIA using oestradiol–isoluminol as the labelled antigen and monoclonal tube antibodies to oestradiol-6-carboxymethyl oxime-BSA passively adsorbed to polystyrene tubes.

2.3.1. Reagents

6-(N-Ethyl-4-[oestradiol-6-(O)-carboxymethyl oxime]-butyl) amino-2,3-dihydrophthalazine-1,4-dione (oestradiol--6-CMO–ABEI conjugate) and monoclonal antibodies to oestradiol-6-CMO–BSA were prepared according to the method of Kim et al. (1982) and kindly donated by Dr F. Kohen, The Department of Hormone Research, The Weizmann Institute of Science, Rehovot, Israel. Polystyrene tubes (Luckham LP3) were coated with monoclonal antibodies (200 μl) as described previously (p. 128). Microperoxidase (MP-11) was obtained from Sigma Chemical Co. Ltd, Poole, Dorset, UK.

The assay buffer (0.1 mol l^{-1}, pH 7.5) is prepared by dissolving 2.5 g $NaH_2PO_4.2H_2O$ plus 11.9 g Na_2HPO_4 in 1 litre of double distilled water containing 1 g of gelatin, 1 g of sodium azide and 9 g of sodium chloride.

Microperoxidase is dissolved in phosphate buffer and the stock solution (1 mg ml^{-1}) stored at 4 °C. The working solution is 20 μg ml^{-1} (50-fold dilution in double distilled water) and is prepared for each assay. This reagent is stable at room temperature for several hours. A working solution (0.3%) of hydrogen peroxide is prepared by diluting an aliquot of stock solution (30%; 100 vol.) 100 times in double distilled water, to give sufficient reagent for the assay and to prime the dispenser before use.

2.3.2. Sample collection and extraction

Blood samples are obtained from women by venepuncture and transferred into tubes containing lithium heparin. After centrifugation the plasma is removed and stored at −20 °C until required. Subsequently, 250 μl of plasma are extracted in duplicate with 2.5 ml of diethyl ether. The aqueous phase is frozen in solid CO_2–ethanol and the organic phase is transferred to a glass tube and evaporated. The dried residues are reconstituted with 500 μl of assay buffer. It is necessary to include duplicate ether blanks in each assay by extracting 250 μl of double distilled water by the same procedure.

2.3.3. Immunoassay procedure

(i) Aliquots of buffer or standard solutions (range 1.95–500 pg per tube) are added in duplicate to assay tubes according to Table 2.

(ii) Oestradiol-6-CMO–ABEI (20 pg per 100 μl of phosphate buffer) is added according to Table 2 and the mixture incubated at 4 °C for 60 min.

Table 2. Solid-phase oestradiol CIA: assay protocol

Assay tube†	Buffer (μl)	Standard or sample (μl)	Tracer (working dilution) (μl)
TR	—	—	100
B_0	100	—	100
Standard or unknown	—	100	100

† TR, Total response tubes; B_0, total binding tubes

(iii) The contents of each tube are aspirated (with the exception of the total response tubes). The tubes (antibody-bound fraction) are washed once by the addition of 1 ml double distilled water to each tube (with the exception of the total response tubes) followed by immediate aspiration.

(iv) Sodium hydroxide (5M, 200 μl) is added to each tube, including the total response tubes; the contents are mixed well and incubated for 60 min at 60 °C.

(v) After cooling to room temperature (NB: 30 min), 100 μl of microperoxidase solution (20 μg ml^{-1}) are added to each individual tube which is immediately placed in the luminometer. (NB: It is not advisable to add microperoxidase to the whole batch of tubes as this reagent is progressively denatured at high pH.)

(vi) Chemiluminescence is initiated by the rapid injection of 100 μl of hydrogen peroxide solution (0.3%) and the signal recorded for 10 sec.

(vii) The unknown values are derived from the dose–response curve (B/B_0, in per cent, versus concentration of oestradiol, in picograms) and multiplied by 18.38 to obtain the results in picomoles per litre (the molecular weight of oestradiol is 272).

2.3.4. Evaluation

A typical dose–response curve and within-batch precision profile are shown in Fig. 4. The sensitivity of the method (defined as the reagent blank minus 2S.D.) is routinely less than 3 pg per tube, which is equivalent to 55.1 pmol l^{-1}. This value is similar to that obtained with a conventional radioimmunoassay (RIA), and may be increased by the analysis of larger volumes of sample or extract. The method gave a mean positive bias of 17% (which was independent of dose over the range 150–1800 pmol l^{-1}) compared to the RIA using polyclonal antiserum, and Dextran-coated charcoal to adsorb the unbound fraction. An estimate of the within-batch precision was obtained by analysing replicate samples from two plasma pools within a single assay (Table 3). The corresponding values of between-batch variation were calculated from the measurement of oestradiol in extracts of two plasma pools used for internal quality control over a period of six months.

Table 3. Solid-phase oestradiol CIA: within- and between-batch precision

	No. of estimates	QC3		QC4	
		Mean	CV (%)	Mean	CV (%)
Intra-assay variation	20	641	8.4	1382	5.4
Inter-assay variation	23	612	10.1	1301	8.3

2.4. Salivary progesterone–direct assay, Immunobead separation

Saliva is a readily accessible body fluid and a variety of RIAs for the assessment of hormonal status have been developed (Landman et al., 1976; Walker et al., 1978; Luisi et al., 1981). In particular, Walker et al. (1981) have developed a method for the measurement of progesterone in order to monitor ovarian function, and a non-isotopic immunoassay has been introduced for the measurement of testosterone (Turkes et al., 1979, 1980).

There are a number of problems associated with the application of immunoassay techniques to the measurement of hormones in saliva which

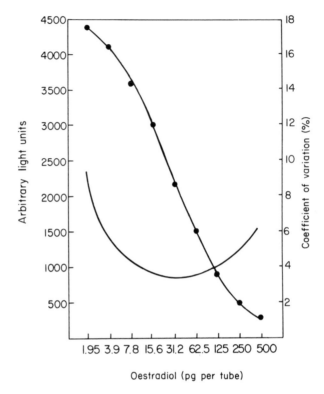

Oestradiol (pg per tube)

Fig. 4. Oestradiol CIA: dose–response curve (●—●) and smoothed precision profile
(——)

include: (i) the extremely low concentrations of the analytes; (ii) the extreme
variability of other components making the material a particularly unsuitable
matrix for direct assays, and (iii) the difficulty of handling fluid which has
degraded on storage. Despite these limitations, we have developed and
evaluated a CIA for the direct measurement of progesterone in 100 μl of
saliva using sheep anti-rabbit IgG covalently linked to polyacrylamide beads
as the solid-phase reagent.

2.4.1. Reagents

Sheep anti-rabbit IgG covalently attached to polyacrylamide beads (Immunobeads) was obtained from Bio-Rad Laboratories, Watford, Herts, UK,
and reconstituted by the addition of 50 ml of assay buffer (0.1 mol l^{-1}
phosphate buffer, pH 7.5) containing 0.1% BSA, 0.9% sodium chloride,
0.1% sodium azide.

2.4.2. Immunoassay procedure

Samples of saliva (3 ml) were collected from healthy female volunteers every morning throughout their complete menstrual cycles and stored at -20 °C until required.

One hundred microlitres of saliva or 100 µl of standard (range 0.76–100 pg progesterone per tube) are added in duplicate to the assay tubes. Subsequently, 100 µl of suitably diluted rabbit anti-progesterone antibody, 100 µl of progesterone-3-CMO–ABEI (30 pg per tube) and 200 µl of immunobead reagent are added and the mixture incubated at 4 °C overnight. Subsequently, 1 ml of phosphate buffer is added to each tube and the contents mixed on a vortex mixer. The tubes are centrifuged (10 min; 2000 g) and the supernatants removed by aspiration. The washing step is repeated. Two hundred microlitres of 2 M sodium hydroxide are added to each tube and the contents incubated at 60 °C for 60 min. After cooling to room temperature, 100 µl of the microperoxidase solution are added to the assay tube, which is placed in the luminometer. The chemiluminescence reaction is initiated and the signal measured for 10 s as described previously. The unknown values are derived from the dose–response curve (B/B_0, in per cent, versus concentration of progesterone, in picograms) and multiplied by 31.7 to obtain the results in picomoles per litre (molecular weight of progesterone is 315).

2.4.3. Evaluation

A dose–response curve and precision profile are shown in Fig. 5. The sensitivity of the method (defined as zero dose minus 2S.D.) is routinely less than 16 pmol l^{-1}. The intra-assay variation at 160 pmol l^{-1} was less than 10%, and the inter-assay variation over 3 months was 18.8%. The concentrations of progesterone (geometric means and ranges) in samples of saliva throughout 14 menstrual cycles as determined by CIA are shown in Fig. 6.

2.5. Direct assays for plasma haptens

The introduction of simple, direct immunoassays for the measurement of steroids in unextracted serum or plasma is one of the most significant advances in steroid methodology for routine clinical application (Ratcliffe, 1983). Extraction with an organic solvent is avoided by the use of reagents which block the binding to, or displace steroids from, serum binding proteins. Other methods involve a change in pH or incubation of the sample at high temperature (Haynes et al., 1980; Al-Dujaili et al., 1981). The measurement of steroids in plasma by a direct assay requires: (i) an antiserum with high avidity and specificity; (ii) a separation technique that reduces misclassification of the label between the antibody-bound and free fractions and, in the case of non-isotopic immunoassay, removes any component that would

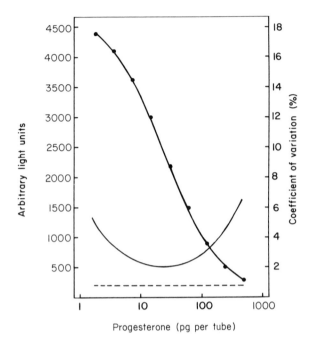

Fig. 5. Progesterone CIA: dose-response curve (●–●) and smoothed precision profile
(——)

enhance or reduce the signal, and (iii) a set of calibrated standards in an
appropriate matrix. To date, direct CIAs have been reported for the
measurement of cortisol (Lindstrom *et al.*, 1982) and progesterone (de
Boever *et al.*, 1984) in plasma, using steroid—isoluminol conjugates.

3.   THE MEASUREMENT OF PROTEINS USING ISOLUMINOL
DERIVATIVES

Several attempts have been made to develop CIAs using proteins (antigens or
antibodies) labelled with derivatives of luminol and isoluminol (Simpson *et
al.*, 1979, 1981). However, the association of luminol with peptides or
proteins significantly lowers the quantum yield. More recent studies (Cheng *et
al.*, 1982; Barnard *et al.*, 1984a; Brockelbank *et al.*, 1984) show that
protein–isoluminol conjugates prepared with a hemisuccinamide derivative of
ABEI (ABEI-H) have acceptable quantum yields upon oxidation at high pH.
Using this derivative, we have prepared human choriogonadotrophin–ABEI

(hCG–ABEI), a non-specific anti-hCG IgG–ABEI and a sheep anti-rabbit IgG–ABEI for use in the development of several CIAs and ICMAs. The stability of each labelled protein is satisfactory, no significant reduction in activity being discerned over 12 months (Brockelbank *et al.*, 1984). Alternative CIAs for the measurement of hCG, luteinizing hormone (LH), follicle-stimulating hormone (FSH) and prolactin have been developed using these protein–isoluminol conjugates. The methods involve the use of: (i) labelled antigens in a competitive assay; (ii) labelled second antibody (i.e. a universal reagent) in a competitive assay, and (iii) labelled first antibody (i.e. a two-site ICMA) in a non-competitive or excess reagent assay.

3.1. Labelled antigen techniques

Competitive binding assays have been developed for the measurement of hCG in serum or urine, and for LH in urine.

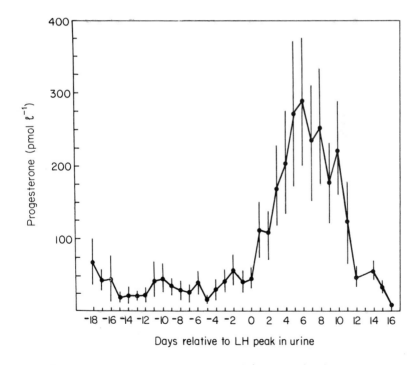

Fig. 6. Salivary progesterone throughout 14 menstrual cycles, mean $\pm$ S.D., $n=14$; lowest to highest mean, 5–100 pg ml^{-1}

3.1.1. Serum or urinary hCG

Early tests for hCG, based upon haemagglutination and latex agglutination have been supplemented with radioimmunoassays (RIAs) in which specific antibodies directed against the β-subunit are capable of detecting pregnancy a few days after implantation (Vaitukaitis et al., 1972). Recently, several RIA kits have become available commercially and have been evaluated (Know et al., 1980). In addition, various non-isotopic immunoassays for the measurement of hCG in serum, plasma, or urine using colorimetry (Tomoda, 1981) or fluorometry (Petterson et al., 1983) have been described. More recently, we developed and evaluated a solid-phase CIA (Barnard et al., 1984a) and assessed its clinical utility for the early detection of pregnancy.

3.1.1.1. Method

The synthesis of the labelled antigen (hCG–ABEI) has been reported (Barnard et al., 1984a). The structure of the protein–isoluminol conjugate is compared with a corresponding steroid derivative in Fig. 7. A flow diagram of the immunoassay is shown in Fig. 8.

3.1.1.2. Evaluation

The method has been evaluated in detail (Barnard et al., 1984a). A typical dose–response curve (mean ± S.D.; $n = 6$) is shown in Fig. 9. The sensitivity of the method (defined as zero dose minus 2S.D.) is $2.0 ± 0.1$ IU l^{-1}, which is essentially similar to the RIA using an iodinated tracer (Amerlex kit; Amersham International, Amersham, Bucks, UK). The concentration of hCG in urine samples from pregnant and non-pregnant women was deter-

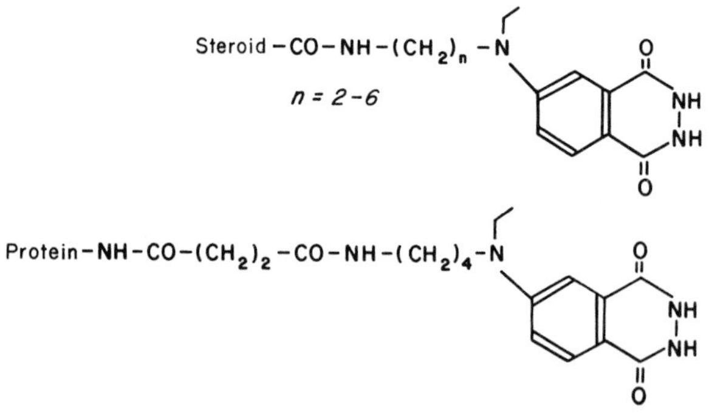

Fig. 7. Structures of chemiluminescent conjugates

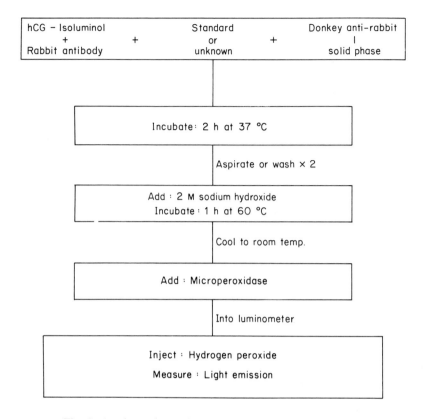

Fig. 8. A schematic outline of solid phase CIA for LH/hCG

mined by CIA and RIA and a comparison of the results is shown in Fig. 10. The CIA had a mean positive bias of 8.1% over the dose range 30–180 IU l^{-1} (the threshold value for pregnancy is 50 IU l^{-1}).

3.1.2. Urinary LH

A practical reference method for the detection of ovulation has involved the measurement of LH by RIA in daily samples of early morning urine (EMU) (Collins *et al.*, 1979). In addition, the collection of urine (every 2–4 h) under carefully controlled conditions has enabled defined changes in the excretion rate of LH (in IU per hour) to be used for predicting the appropriate time for oocyte recovery prior to extracorporeal fertilisation (Edwards *et al.*, 1982). These authors used a semi-quantitative haemagglutination immunoassay for the immediate prediction of ovulation, which involved the use of microtitre

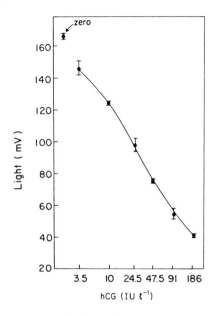

Fig. 9. hCG CIA: dose–response curve

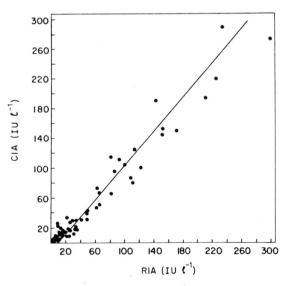

Fig. 10. Correlation between CIA and RIA for the measurement of hCG: $n=60$; $r=0.98$

plates and the serial dilution of each urine sample. Recently we reported a quantitative CIA for the measurement of urinary LH (Brockelbank *et al.*, 1984). The method was assessed for sensitivity, precision, bias, parallelism and long-term quality control.

3.1.2.1. Immunoassay procedure

The synthesis of the labelled antigen and the immunoassay procedure have been reported (Brockelbank *et al.*, 1984). A flow diagram of the method is shown in Fig. 8.

3.1.2.2. Evaluation

The minimum concentration of LH that could be significantly distinguished from zero (mean $-$ 2S.D.) was calculated from six dose–response curves. The value (mean $\pm$ S.D.) was 0.2 ± 0.1 IU l^{-1}. An estimate of the intra-assay precision was obtained by analysing 20 replicate samples from four EMUs (mean doses 17.1, 51.4, 193.1 and 437.9 IU l^{-1}) within a single assay. The coefficients of variation were 25.7, 9.7, 8.4 and 9.0% respectively. In addition, an assessment of long-term quality control of the assay was obtained (over 18 months) by the accumulation of data from 6 parameters. The`results are shown in Table 4. The method has been used to identify the peak excretion of LH as a reference point for dating events during the ovarian cycle.

Table 4. Solid-phase urinary LH CIA: long-term quality control

Variable	No. of batches	Mean	S.D.	CV (%)
Total light yield (mV)	40	35.94	4.82	13.4
Total binding (B_0, mV)	40	11.86	1.09	9.2
Analyte conc. 50% inhibition (IU l^{-1})	40	67.0	7.0	10.4
Non-specific binding (mV)	40	1.74	0.47	27.0
Quality control, sample 1 (IU l^{-1})	40	57.0	10.5	18.4
Quality control, sample 2 (IU l^{-1})	40	207.5	16.4	7.9

Reference range 30–300 IU l^{-1}

3.2. Labelled antibody techniques

A labelled antibody can be used as a universal reagent in a competitive binding assay, or as a specific or universal label in an immunometric assay.

3.2.1. Competitive binding assays

The availability of sheep anti-rabbit IgG reagent labelled with ABEI (Cheng et al. 1982) has enabled the development of CIAs for hCG, LH, FSH and prolactin. The principle of these assays depends upon the immobilization of a limiting concentration of antigen on an appropriate solid phase (plastic tube, polyacrylamide beads or cellulose). Specific rabbit antibody, sample or standard and excess labelled antibody are added to the tubes and the mixture is incubated at 37 °C for 2 h. The reaction mixture is aspirated (coated tube), or centrifuged and aspirated (particulate solid phase). The antibody-bound fraction is washed, incubated in the presence of sodium hydroxide at 60 °C and chemiluminescence is initiated. A schematic outline of this approach is shown in Fig. 11. To date, the limited availability of the antigens restricts the application of this approach.

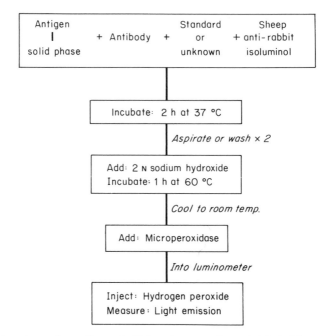

Fig. 11. A schematic outline of CIA using a universal label (sheep anti-rabbit IgG–isoluminol)

3.2.2. Immunochemiluminometric assay

In 1968, Miles and Hales introduced an important new type of immunoassay which they termed immunoradiometric assay (IRMA), based on the use of isotopically labelled antibodies. In the basic form, excess labelled antibody is added to bind all the antigen. Subsequently, the antigen-bound and free fractions are separated and the radioactivity determined in the bound fraction, which is directly proportional to the total amount of antigen present. The advantages of an excess reagent system are shorter incubation times, greater sensitivity and a wider working range of analyte (Jackson *et al.*, 1983).

In addition, two-site IRMAs have been developed for compounds with more than one antigenic determinant (epitope), which involve the immobilization of excess specific antibody on a solid phase (Miles, 1977). The samples containing analyte are added and after incubation the phases are separated. A second antibody of different specificity, labelled with radioisotope, is added in excess. After incubation, the reaction mixture is removed and the amount of label remaining in the assay tube is directly proportional to the concentration of analyte. The differences between RIA and IRMA have been discussed (see Chapter 5 in this volume). Non-isotopic immunometric assays have been developed and include immunoenzymometric assay (Gnemmi *et al.*, 1978), immunofluorometric assay (Smith *et al.*, 1981) and more recently, immunochemiluminometric assay (ICMA; Cheng *et al.*, 1982; Schroeder *et al.*, 1981; Weeks *et al.*, 1983a,b,c, 1984). In addition, we have developed and evaluated an ICMA for the measurement of hCG in urine (Barnard *et al.*, 1984a).

3.2.2.1. Serum or urinary hCG

The preparation of antibodies labelled with isoluminol and the antibody-coated tubes has been described previously (Barnard *et al.*, 1984a). A schematic outline of the immunoassay procedure is shown in Fig. 12.

3.2.2.1.1. Evaluation

A dose–response curve and precision profile are shown in Fig. 13. The minimum concentration of hCG that could be significantly distinguished from zero (mean $-$ 2S.D.) ranged from 1.8 ± 0.4 IU l^{-1} (2 h incubation) to 0.25 ± 0.05 IU l^{-1} (7 day incubation). It is apparent that shorter incubation times could be used with improved monoclonal antibodies (Barnard *et al.*, 1984b). The intra-assay precision was 7.9% (dose 30.5 IU l^{-1}). The inter-assay CV (six assays) of the same quality control sample was 18.4%. The concentration of hCG, determined in selected samples of urine from pregnant and non-pregnant women by ICMA (y) and RIA (x) correlated well: $r = 0.97$, $n = 64$; $y = 0.978x + 0.63$. The incidence of positive and negative results (with a cut-off value of 50 IU l^{-1}) was the same for both tests.

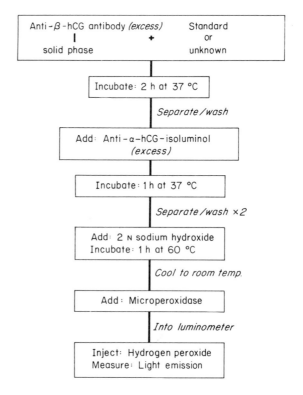

Fig. 12. A schematic outline of ICMA for the measurement of hCG

3.3. The limitations of current isoluminol derivatives

Several successful attempts have been made to develop CIAs with the use of proteins (antigens or antibodies) labelled with derivatives of luminol and isoluminol. Although these conjugates have been shown to be extremely stable (Brockelbank *et al.*, 1984), they have a relatively low quantum yield. Consequently, for high sensitivity, the end-point measurement is preceded by an incubation at high temperature and alkaline pH. The incubation with sodium hydroxide before oxidation facilitates the dissociation of the anti-body-bound complex and may well break up the labelled antigen by alkaline hydrolysis resulting the release of the chemiluminescent moiety. Consequent-ly, the conditions for each assay must be optimized in terms of temperature, time and the concentration of sodium hydroxide. The synthesis of new derivatives of isoluminol that are more easily dissociated from their protein moiety will increase quantum yields of chemiluminescence on oxidation without prolonged incubation under these conditions. In addition, alternative

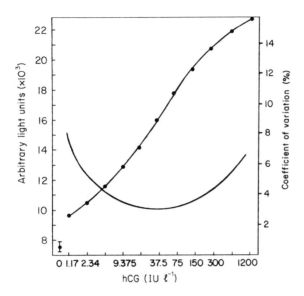

Fig. 13. hCG ICMA: dose–response curve (●—●) and smoothed precision profile (——)

techniques to enhance sensitivity are being investigated. It is envisaged that CIAs using alternative isoluminol labels will be available in the near future that combine the advantage of high stability with ease of oxidation. At present we add the last reagent (i.e. hydrogen peroxide) by rapid injection when the assay tube is situated in front of the photo-detector, because the rate of the chemiluminescent reaction is too fast for the reagent to be added outside of the instrument. Alternative oxidation systems that lead to constant, stable light emissions (cf. bioluminescent reactions) might be preferable.

4. ACRIDINIUM ESTERS

In 1981, Simpson et al. reported the use of acridinium esters as labels in immunoassays. The use of these compounds may increase quantum efficiency, avoid serious quenching when labels are associated with proteins or haptens, and allow simpler oxidation systems involving alkaline peroxide alone. A comparison of the end-point determination of acridinium and isoluminol conjugates is shown in Fig. 14. In the reports of assays with protein–acridinium conjugates (Weeks et al., 1983a,b), the most highly active conjugates of protein and acridinium ester have yielded greater specific activities than those obtained from the equivalent ^{125}I-labelled proteins and

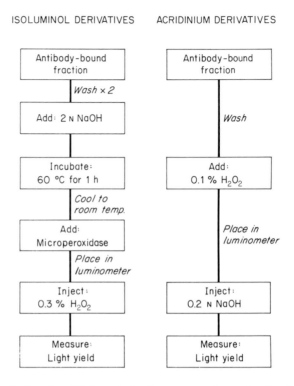

Fig. 14. Isoluminol and acridinium derivatives: comparison of end-point determination

are stable for at least 11 months when stored at −20 °C. Currently, we have developed and are evaluating an ICMA for the measurement of hCG with protein–acridinium derivatives (Barnard *et al.*, 1984b).

4.1. Immunochemiluminometric assay of hCG

The synthesis of 4-(2-succinimidyloxycarbonylethyl)phenyl-10-methylacridinium-9-carboxylate fluorosulphonate has been reported (Weeks *et al.*, 1983b), and the structure is shown in comparison with the corresponding isoluminol derivative in Fig. 15. The activated acridinium ester was kindly donated by Dr Iraj Beheshti of the School of Molecular Sciences, University of Sussex, Falmer, UK. Acridinium-labelled anti-β-hCG antibodies were prepared according to the method of Weeks *et al.*, (1983b). Polystyrene tubes coated with excess monoclonal anti-α-hCG antibodies were kindly donated by Dr Nick Slocum, Monoclonal Antibodies Inc., High Wycombe, Bucks., UK. Monoclonal antibodies to β-hCG were kindly donated by Dr Fortune

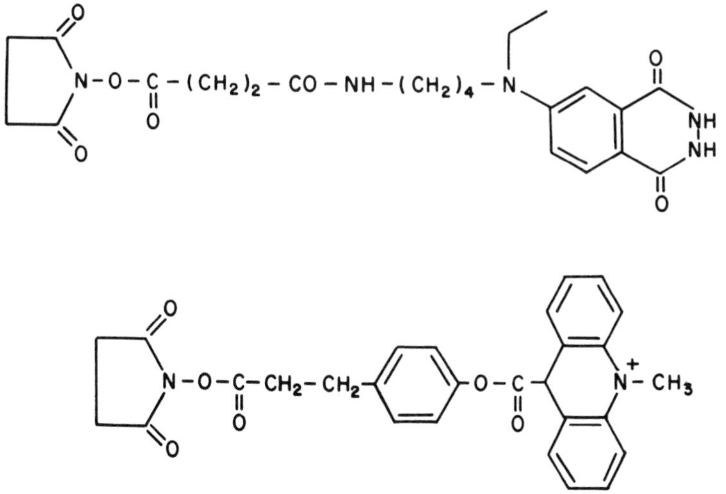

Fig. 15. The proposed structures of activated esters of (a) isoluminol and (b) acridine derivatives

Kohen, Department of Hormone Research, The Weizmann Institute of Science, Rehovot, Israel.

4.1.1. Assay procedure

An outline of the method is shown in Fig. 16. Fifty microlitres of plasma or 50 μl of standard (range 0–320 IU l^{-1} of assay buffer) are added in duplicate to the anti-α-hCG antibody-coated tubes. After an incubation of 10 min at room temperature, the contents of the tube are removed by aspiration. One hundred microlitres of suitably diluted (excess) anti-β-hCG IgG–acridinium conjugate are added and the mixture incubated at room temperature for 30 min. Subsequently, the contents are removed by aspiration and 500 μl of phosphate buffer are added to each tube and aspirated. This washing step is repeated twice. Two hundred microlitres of 0.1% hydrogen peroxide in double distilled water are added to the assay tube, which is placed in the luminometer. The chemiluminescence reaction is initiated by the rapid injection of 100 μl of 0.2 M sodium hydroxide and the signal measured for 10 s, as described previously. The unknown values are derived from the dose–response curve (B/B_0, in per cent, versus concentration of hCG, in IU per litre).

An analogue dose–response curve is shown in Fig. 17. The minimum concentration of hCG that could be significantly distinguished from zero

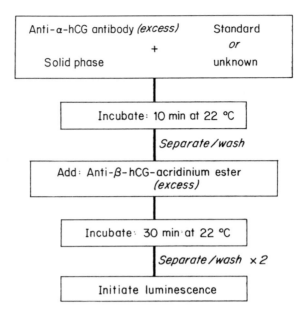

Fig. 16. A schematic outline of ICMA for the measurement of hCG using an acridinium ester derivative

(mean − 2S.D.) was 0.9 ± 0.1 IU l^{-1}. The value could be increased by an order of magnitude if the incubation time with the capture antibody was increased to 1 h. The method is being evaluated in detail.

4.2. Chemiluminescence immunoassay of progesterone

Recently, we have developed and evaluated a solid-phase CIA for the measurement of progesterone in extracts of peripheral plasma using a novel hapten–acridinium ester conjugate, 11α-progesteryl N-succininoyl tyramine 4-(N'-methyl) acridinium-9-carboxylate (Richardson *et al.*, 1984). The sensitivity and precision of the method are similar to those obtained by a CIA using progesterone-11α-succinyl-ABEI as the label. A carefully selected monoclonal antibody is used to minimize method bias. The mean value over the dose range 3–42 nmol l^{-1} is −8.4%.

4.3. The advantages and disadvantages of acridinium esters

Various acridinium salts can be stimulated to produce light in the presence of dilute alkaline hydrogen peroxide in the absence of a catalyst (McCapra, 1974). Such compounds include derivatives of acridine possessing a quaternary nitrogen centre which can be derivatized to produce a labile phenyl ester. The chemiluminescent reaction involves the hydrolysis of the ester bond, intermediate dioxetenone production by hydroperoxide ions and the formation of electronically excited N-methylacridone. Consequently, the chemiluminescent moiety is liberated from hapten or protein prior to electronic excitation. This reaction minimizes quenching from the sample and results in the restoration of a relatively high quantum yield without resort to more complicated chemical hydrolytic procedures. Thus the oxidation reaction is relatively simple and cheap.

Nevertheless, there are certain disadvantages. The presence of the phenyl ester bond, an essential feature of the chemiluminescent species, results in a

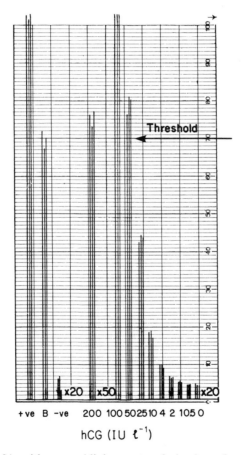

Fig. 17. hCG ICMA with an acridinium ester derivative of anti-hCG: analogue dose–response curve with the results from three pregnancy tests (+ve, positive; B, borderline; −ve, negative). Threshold value, 48 IU 1^{-1}; ×20, ×50 attenuator settings on chart recorder

conjugate that is inherently unstable. In addition, in aqueous solution, acridinium esters exist in equilibrium with their corresponding pseudo-bases (Zaklika, 1976). High pH immunoassay buffers favour pseudo-base formation and it is usually necessary to reform the quaternary nitrogen by the addition of acid prior to oxidation by base (Weeks et al., 1983b). In particular, this is an essential feature of the progesterone CIA. Moreover, storage of the conjugates at higher pH than 6.3 is not recommended due to the occurrence of a dark-reaction with concomitant loss of chemiluminescent activity (Zaklika, 1976). At the present time, another impediment to the development of CIAs with acridinium esters is the absence of a commercially available stable derivative.

5.   FUTURE DEVELOPMENTS

The results to date show that derivatives of isoluminol and acridinium esters are useful alternatives to isotopic labels for the measurement of haptens in diluted biological fluids or in concentrated extracts and for the measurement of proteins in plasma or urine. The use of enhancers in place of sodium hydroxide will make the isoluminol methods easier and quicker to perform. Similarly, the increasing availability of acridinium derivatives may facilitate the introduction of immunoassays that are significantly more sensitive than RIAs or IRMAs with iodinated antigens and antibodies (Weeks et al., 1984). In addition, we envisage the introduction of immunometric assays for haptens as well as proteins. Currently, we are developing direct immunochemiluminometric assays for oestradiol and progesterone in unextracted serum and saliva.

Although there are luminometers available commercially, there is still the need to design and develop two types of instrument that are purpose-built for CIAs and ICMAs. The first type would be a simple, single-tube instrument that can be powered by a dry battery and would be appropriate for clinic or home use. This development would extend the availability of relatively sophisticated clinically useful tests to the doctor's surgery or enable a patient to monitor their own treatment. These simple instruments would be used in association with the appropriate reagent presentation (e.g. reagent strips or lyophilized pellets). The legislative and emotive bias against the use of radioisotopes outside specially equipped laboratories precludes the use of isotopic labels for this purpose. Moreover, the problems associated with the use of radioactivity are pertinent to the developing countries where it may be inappropriate or impossible to institute or maintain a high degree of sophistication in clinical chemistry, but where the needs are perhaps more urgent. The second type of instrument would be more complex, with a capacity of several hundred tubes (e.g. the Berthold Auto-biolumat). This luminometer is similar to existing solid and liquid scintillation counters although an additional module is required to inject the oxidant. The availability of this type of instrument would facilitate the acceptance of CIA in those countries where RIA is well established.

The techniques described in this report involve rapid kinetics and necessitate the precise injection of oxidant into the tube, which is positioned in front of the photo-detector. More recently, we have developed a bioluminescence immunoassay and an immunobioluminometric assay for the measurement of hCG using glucose 6-phosphate dehydrogenase and bacterial bioluminescence monitoring reagents (Kohen et al., 1984). The continuous light emission obtained from these sensitive immunoassays has obviated the need for an injection system. Light detection may be performed in existing luminometers or liquid scintillation counters. Alternatively, we envisage that these methods may be used in association with dipstick or microtitre plate luminescence photometers.

ACKNOWLEDGEMENTS

The investigators received financial support from the King's Voluntary Research Trust, the Medical Research Council and Wallac Oy, Turku, Finland. We gratefully acknowledge the contributions to this work of Professor W. P. Collins, Dr Fortune Kohen, Professor F. McCapra, Dr I. Beheshti, Mr A. Richardson and colleagues from the Department of Obstetrics and Gynaecology, King's College School of Medicine and Dentistry.

REFERENCES

Al-Dujaili, E. A. S., Williams, B. C. and Edwards, C. R. W. (1981). The development and application of a direct radioimmunoassay for corticosterone. Steroids, **37**, 157–176.

Anderson, J. M. Faini, G. J. and Wampler, J. E. (1978). Construction of instrumentation for bioluminescence and chemiluminescence. Meth. Enzymol. **57**, 529–540.

Barnard, G., Collins, W. P., Kohen, F. and Lindner, H. R. (1981). A preliminary study of the measurement of urinary pregnanediol-3α-glucuronide by a solid-phase chemiluminescence immunoassay. In Bioluminescence and Chemiluminescence: Basic Chemistry and Analytical Applications (M. DeLuca and W. D. McElroy, eds), Academic Press, New York, pp. 311–317.

Barnard, G., Kim, J. B., Brockelbank, J. L., Collins, W. P., Kohen, F. and Gaier, B. (1984a). The measurement of choriogonadotropin by chemiluminescence immunoassay and immunochemiluminometric assay. 1. Use of isoluminol derivatives. Clin. Chem., **30**, 538–541.

Barnard, G., Brockelbank, J. L., Kim, J. B. and Collins, W. P. (1984b). The use of isoluminol and acridinium labels in immunoassay. In Analytical Applications of Bioluminescence and Chemiluminescence (L. J. Kricka, P. E. Stanley, G. H. G. Thorpe and T. P. Whitehead, eds), Academic Press, New York, pp. 159–162.

Brockelbank, J. L., Barnard, G., Kim, J. B., Collins, W. P., Kohen, F. and Geier, B. (1984). The measurement of urinary LH by a solid-phase chemiluminescence immunoassay. *Ann. Clin. Biochem.*, **21**, 284–289.

Cheng, P-J., Hemmilä, I. and Lövgren, T. (1982). Development of solid-phase immunoassay using chemiluminescent IgG conjugates. *J. Immunol. Meth.*, **48**, 159–168.

Collins, W. P., Collins, P. O., Kilpatrick, M. J., Manning, P. A., Pike, J. and Tyler, J. P. P. (1979). The concentrations of urinary oestrone-3-glucuronide, LH and pregnanediol-3α-glucuronide as indices of ovarian function. *Acta Endocr., Copenh.* **93**, 123–128.

Collins, W. P., Barnard, G. J. R., Kim, J. B., Weerasekera, D. W., Kohen, F., Lindner, H. R. and Eshhar, Z. (1983). Chemiluminescence immunoassay of plasma steroids and urinary steroid glucuronides. In *Immunoassays for Clinical Chemistry* (W. M. Hunter and J. E. T. Corrie, eds), Churchill Livingstone, Edinburgh, pp. 373–379.

de Boever, J., Kohen, F, Vanderkerckhove, D. and Van Maede, G. (1984). Solid-phase chemiluminescence immunoassay for progesterone in unextracted serum. *Clin. Chem.* **30**, 1637–1641.

Edwards, R. G., Anderson, G., Pickering, J. and Purdy, J. M. (1982). Rapid assay of urinary LH in women using a simplified method of Hi-gonavis. In *Human Conception* in vitro (R. G. Edwards and J. M. Purdy, eds), Academic Press, London, pp. 19–34.

Gnemmi, E., O'Sullivan, M. J., Chieregatti, G., Simmons, M., Simmonds, A., Bridges, J. W. and Marks, V. (1978). A sensitive immunoenzymometric assay (IEMA) to quantitate hormones and drugs. In *Enzyme Labelled Immunoassay of Hormones and Drugs* (S. B. Pal, ed.), Walter de Gruyter, New York, pp. 29–41.

Haynes, S. P., Corcoran, J. M., Eastman, C. J. and Doy, F. A. (1980). Radioimmunoassay of progesterone in unextracted serum. *Clin. Chem.* **26**, 1607–1609.

Jackson, T. M., Marshall, N. J. and Ekins, R. P. (1983). Optimization of immunoradiometric (labelled antibody) assays. In *Immunoassays for Clinical Chemistry* (W. M. Hunter and J. E. T. Corrie, eds), Churchill Livingstone, Edinburgh, pp. 557–575.

Kim, J. B. (1983). The development of chemiluminescence immunoassays for the measurement of plasma steroids and urinary steroid glucuronides. PhD thesis, University of London.

Kim, J. B., Barnard, G. J., Collins, W. P., Kohen, F., Lindner, H. R. and Eshhar, Z. (1982). Measurement of plasma estradiol-17β by solid-phase chemiluminescence immunoassay. *Clin. Chem.*, **28**, 1120–1124.

Know, B. S., McKee, J. W. A., Hair, P. I. and France, J. (1980). Determination of β-choriogonadotrophin in human plasma: evaluation and comparison of five 'kit' methods. *Clin. chem.*, **26**, 1890–1895.

Kohen, F., Pazzagli, M., Kim, J. B. and Lindner, H. R. (1979). An assay procedure for plasma progesterone based on antibody-enhanced chemiluminescence. *FEBS Lett.* **104**, 201–205.

Kohen, F., Kim, J. B., Barnard, G. and Lindner, H. R. (1980a). An assay for urinary estriol-16α-glucuronide based on antibody-enhanced chemiluminescence. *Steroids*, **36**, 405–419.

Kohen, F., Pazzagli, M., Kim, J. B. and Lindner, H. R. (1980b). An immunoassay for plasma cortisol based on chemiluminescence. *Steroids*, **36**, 421–437.

Kohen, F., Bayer, E., Wilchek, M., Barnard, G., Kim, J. B., Collins, W. P., Beheshti, I., Richardson, A. and McCapra, F. (1984). The development of luminescence-based immunoassays. In *Applications of Bioluminescence and Chemiluminescence* (L. J. Kricka ed), Academic Press, New York, pp. 149–158.

Landman, A. D., Sanford, L. M., Howland, B. E., Dawes, C. and Pritchard, E. T. (1976). Testosterone in human saliva. *Experimentia*, **32**, 940.

Lindstrom, L., Meurling, L. and Lovgren, T. (1982). The measurement of serum cortisol by a solid-phase chemiluminescence immunoassay. *J. Steroid Biochem.*, **16**, 577–580.

Luisi, M., Franchi, F., Kicovic, P. M., Silvestri, D., Cossu, G., Catarsi, A. L., Barletta, D. and Gasperi, G. (1981). Radioimmunoassay for progesterone in human saliva during the menstrual cycle. *J. Steroid Biochem.*, **14**, 1060–1074.

McCapra, F. (1974). Chemiluminescence of organic compounds. *Prog. Org. Chem.*, **8**, 231–277.

Miles, L. E. M. (1977). Immunoradiometric assay (IRMA) and two site IRMA system (assay of soluble antigens using labelled antibodies). In *Handbook of Radioimmunoassay* (G. E. Abraham, ed.), Dekker, New York, pp. 131–178.

Miles, L. E. M. and Hales, C. N. (1968). Labelled antibodies and immunological assay systems. *Nature, Lond.* **219**, 186–189.

Petterson, K., Siitari, H., Hemmilä, I., Soini, E., Lovgren, T., Hanninen, V., Tanner, P. and Stenman, U.-H. (1983). Time-resolved fluoroimmunoassay of human choriogonadotropin. *Clin. Chem.*, **29**, 60–64.

Ratcliffe, W. A. (1983) Direct (non-extraction) serum assays for steroids. In *Immunoassays for Clinical Chemistry* (W. M. Hunter and J. E. T. Corrie, eds), Churchill Livingstone, Edinburgh, pp. 401–409.

Richardson, A., Kim, J. B., Barnard, G., Collins, W. P. and McCapra, F. (1985). Chemiluminescence immunoassay of plasma progesterone using progesterone-acridinium ester as the labelled antigen. *Clin. Chem.* in press.

Seliger, H. H. (1978). Excited states and absolute calibrations in chemiluminescence. *Meth. Enzymol.* **57**, 560–600.

Schroeder, H. R., Vogelhut, P. O., Carrico, R. J., Boguslaski, R. C. and Buckler, R. T. (1976). Competitive protein-binding assay for biotin monitored by chemiluminescence. *Analyt. Chem.*, **48**, 1933–1937.

Schroeder, H. R., Hines, C. M., Osborn, D. D., Moore, R. P., Hurtle, R. L., Wotoman, F. F., Rogers, R. W. and Vogelhut, P. O. (1981). Immunochemiluminometric assay for hepatitis B surface antigen. *Clin. Chem.* **27**, 1378–1384.

Simpson, J. S. A., Campbell, A. M., Ryall, M. E. T. and Woodhead, J. S. (1979). A stable chemiluminescence-labelled antibody for immunological assays. *Nature, Lond.* **274**, 646–647.

Simpson, J. S. A., Campbell, A. K., Woodhead, J. S., Richardson, A., Hart, R. and McCapra, F. (1981). Chemiluminescence labels in immunoassay. In *Bioluminescence and Chemiluminescence: Basic Chemistry and Analytical Applications*. (M. DeLuca and W. D. McElroy, eds), Academic Press, New York, pp. 673–679.

Smith, D. S., Al-Hakiem, H. H. and Landon, J. (1981). A review of fluoroimmunoassay and immunofluorometric assay. *Ann. Clin. Biochem.*, **18**, 253–274.

Tomoda, S. (1981). Enzyme immunoassay for human chorionic gonadotrophin and its clinical application. *Acta Obstet. Gynaecol. jap.*, **33**, 1085–1089.

Turkes, A., Turkes, A. O., Joyce, B. G., Read, G. F. and Riad-Fahmy, D. (1979). A sensitive solid-phase enzymeimmunoassay for testosterone in plasma and saliva. *Steroids* **33**, 347–359.

Turkes, A. O., Turkes, A., Joyce, B. G. and Riad-Fahmy, D. (1980). A sensitive enzymeimmunoassay with a fluorimetric end-point for the determination of testosterone in female plasma and saliva. *Steroids* **35**, 89–101.

Vaitukaitis, J. L., Braunstein, G. D. and Ross, G. T. (1972). A radioimmunoassay which specifically measures human chorionic gonadotrophin in the presence of human luteinising hormone. *Am. J. Obstet. Gynec.* **113**, 751–758.

Walker, R. F., Riad-Fahmy, D. and Read, G. F. (1978). Adrenal status assessed by direct radioimmunoassay of cortisol in whole saliva or parotid fluid. *Clin. Chem.* **24**, 1460–1463.

Walker, S., Mustafa, A., Walker, R. F. and Riad-Fahmy, D. (1981). The role of salivary progesterone in studies of infertile women. *Br. J. Obstet. Gynaecol.*, **88**, 1009–1015.

Weeks, I., McCapra, F., Campbell, A. K. and Woodhead, J. S. (1983a). Immunoassays using chemiluminescent labelled antibodies. In *Immunoassays for Clinical Chemistry* (W. M. Hunter and J. E. T. Corrie, eds), Churchill Livingstone, Edinburgh, pp. 525–530.

Weeks, I., Beheshti, I., McCapra, F., Campbell, A. K. and Woodhead, J. S. (1983b). Acridinium esters as high-specific activity labels in immunoassay. *Clin. Chem.* **29**, 1474–1479.

Weeks, I., Campbell, A. K. and Woodhead, J. S. (1983c). Two-site immunochemiluminometric assay (ICMA) for human α_1-fetoprotein. *Clin. Chem.* **29**, 1480–1483.

Weeks, I., Sturgess, M., Siddle, K. Jones, M. K. and Woodhead, J. S. (1984). A high sensitivity immunochemiluminometric assay for human thyrotrophin. *Clin. Endocrinol.* **20**, 489–495.

Weerasekera, D. A., Kim, J. B., Barnard, G. J. and Collins, W. P. (1983). The measurement of serum thyroxine by solid-phase chemiluminescence immunoassay. *Ann. Clin. Biochem.* **20**, 100–104.

Zaklika, K. A. (1976). Reaction mechanisms in chemiluminescesce. DPhil thesis, University of Sussex.

Alternative Immunoassays
Edited by W. P. Collins
© 1985 John Wiley & Sons Ltd

CHAPTER 10

Chemiluminescence energy transfer: a technique for homogeneous immunoassay

A.K. Campbell, P. A. Roberts and A. Patel

Department of Medical Biochemistry,
Welsh National School of Medicine,
Heath Park, Cardiff CF4 4XN, UK

1. INTRODUCTION

Walk out on to a beach at night and you may be lucky enough to find a range of organisms which glow in the dark. These luminous species may include continuously glowing bacteria on a dying invertebrate or a decaying fish, a flashing syllid worm on a piece of green seaweed, or a hydroid colony lurking under a stone, luminescing as you stroke it. One such hydroid of world-wide distribution is *Obelia geniculata* (Fig. 1), found most commonly growing in large colonies on brown seaweeds. This organism contains a photoprotein, obelin, which emits blue light (λ_{max} 475 nm) when it binds calcium (Campbell, 1974). Yet the organism, or vesicles isolated from it (Campbell and Hallett, 1978), emit bluish-green light (λ_{max} 508 nm), with a much sharper spectrum. The cause of this spectral shift is a green fluorescent protein in the same cells as obelin, observable under a fluorescent microscope (Fig. 1). It was while studying this phenomenon of chemiluminescence energy transfer using a dual wavelength luminometer (Fig. 2, Table 1) at the Marine Biological Association Laboratory, Plymouth, during the summers of 1974, 1975, 1976 and 1977, that we realized that a similar principle could potentially provide a very sensitive method for quantifying ligand–ligand interactions, such as antibody–antigen binding (Fig. 3), without the need for separation of bound and free ligand (Campbell et al., 1980; Hallett and Campbell, 1982a).

153

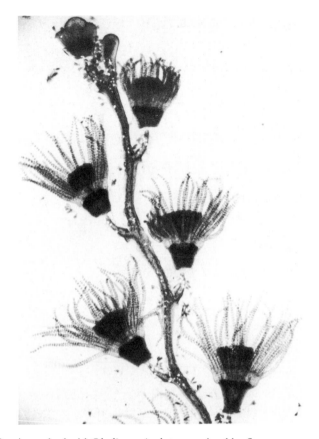

Fig. 1. The luminous hydroid *Obelia geniculata* examined by fluorescence microscopy: fluorescent spots represent luminous cells containing green fluorescent protein

But before considering the application of chemiluminescence energy transfer to immunoassay let us first examine the need for homogeneous (non-separation) immunoassay and the previously reported methods for achieving this objective.

2. THE NEED FOR HOMOGENEOUS IMMUNOASSAY

Ever since the establishment of heterogeneous immunoassays, namely those requiring separation of bound and free antigen or antibody, by Berson and Yalow (1959) and their subsequent development in the 1960s, several groups of workers have attempted to remove the need for this separation step. Such non-separation assays, where all the reagents plus sample are contained in one tube and then analysed, are known as homogeneous immunoassays and have four major advantages. Firstly, the separation step introduces inaccura-

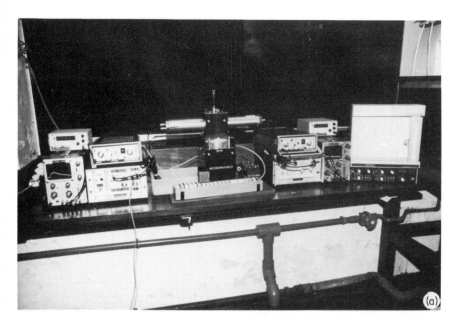

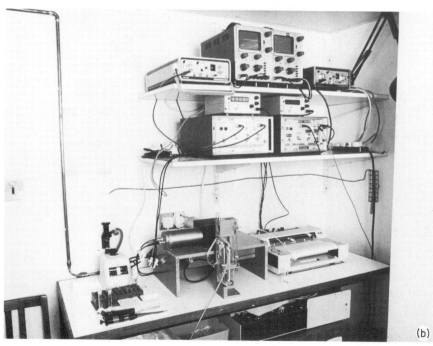

Fig. 2. Dual wavelength luminometers: (a) photomultiplier tubes opposite each other; (b) photomultiplier tubes at right angles to minimize detection of light scattering from the other filter

Table 1. Energy transfer in *Obelia geniculata*

Sample	Ratio of chemiluminescence at 509 and 470 nm
(a) Organisms	
Obelia geniculata (hydroid)	7.81 ± 0.46
Obelia lucifera (medusa)	2.44 ± 0.23
Phialidium hemisphericum (medusa) †	0.71 ± 0.07
(b) Vesicles	
Lumisomes isolated from *Obelia geniculata*	2.23
Lumisomes + triton	1.00
(c) Isolated photoprotein	
Homogenized *Obelia geniculata*	1.03 ± 0.06
Purified obelin	0.95 ± 0.03

Measurements were made using a dual wavelength luminometer [Fig. 2(a)]. Values were corrected for the spectral sensitivity of the two photomultiplier tubes and the transmission of the filters. Organisms (a) were stimulated with 1 ml of artificial sea water (Na^+ replaced by K^+). Vesicles (b) were stimulated by adding 1 ml of artificial sea water. Free obelin (c) was stimulated by adding 0.5 ml of 50 mM $CaCl_2$ to a suspension in 0.1 M Tris + 0.1 mM EDTA pH 7.4.

† No green fluorescence or energy transfer was detactable in the *Phialidium* specimens at Plymouth. This is in contrast to reports of other species of *Phialidium* (Morin, 1974; Levine and Ward, 1982)

cy, and is laborious and expensive, complicating automated assays. Secondly, the measurement of free hormones and drugs is best carried out by homogeneous assays which do not significantly disturb the equilibrium between bound and free antigen in the biological sample. Thirdly, a change in the nature of the signal of the label when bound to antibody (e.g. a wavelength shift) can circumvent some of the problems of 'competition' type assays, limited normally by the affinity of the antibody. A homogeneous method would enable rapidly dissociating ligands, such as cell surface receptors and enzymes, to be used as binding proteins. Fourthly, a major problem in cell biology is the difficulty of measuring chemical changes within living cells. The study of intracellular free calcium (Ashley and Campbell, 1979; Campbell *et al.*, 1979; Hallett and Campbell, 1982a; Campbell, 1983) and oxygen radicals (Campbell *et al.*, 1984) has highlighted the importance of such measurements. Homogeneous immunoassays for metabolites such as cyclic AMP or hormones would enable the mechanisms underlying cell activation and cell injury to be studied in single, living cells.

The first study of antibody–antigen binding without a separation step was carried out by Arquilla and Stavitsky in 1956 using erythrocyte-labelled insulin to detect insulin antibodies in diabetics. The first homogeneous immunoassay was established, for penicillin, by measuring a change in fluorescence polarization when fluorescein-labelled penicillin bound to its antibody (Dandliker and Feigen, 1961). The advent of electron spin resonance (ESR) labels enabled a similar change in rotational correlation to be used to establish a homogeneous immunoassay for morphine (Leute et al., 1972). The application of enzyme, fluorescent and chemiluminescent labels has led to the development of many homogeneous immunoassays for a range of haptens and protein antigens (Table 2). These can be classified on the basis

Table 2. Some examples of homogeneous immunoassay

Basis	Type (see Table 3)	Analyte	Reference
Enzyme inhibition	A1+B1(a)	Drugs and proteins	Rubenstein et al. (1972); Crowl et al. (1980); Gibbons et al. (1980)
Fluorescence quenching	A2+B1(a)	HSA, HIgG, HPL	Nargessi & Landon (1981)
Fluorescence quenching	A2+B1(b)	DNP	Velick et al. (1960)
Fluorescence enhancement	A2+B1(c)	T4	Smith (1977)
Fluorescent substrate	A2+B1(a)	Drugs, IgG	Burd (1981)
Fluorescence excitation energy transfer	A2+B1(b) or B1(a)	T4, drugs, Ig, C3, various proteins	Ullman et al. (1976); Lim et al. (1980); Ullman and Khanna (1981)
Fluorescence polarization	A3+B1d	Penicillin	Dandliker and Feigen (1961)
Chemiluminescence quenching or enhancement	A4+B1(a), (b)or(c)	Biotin, progesterone	Schroeder et al. (1976b); Kohen et al. (1979); Pazzagli et al. (1982)
Chemiluminescence energy transfer	A4+B2(a)	Cyclic AMP, IgG, C9, progesterone	Patel et al. (1983); Patel and Campbell (1983); Campbell and Patel (1983)
Change in ESR	A5+B2(b)	Morphine	Leute et al. (1972)
Formation of immune complexes (rate nephelometry)	A6+B1(d)	IgG, IgA, α_1-anti-trypsin, C9	Sternberg (1977); Carr, I., Fifield, R. Morgan B. P. and A. K. Campbell, (unpublished)
Liposome lyses inhibition	A1 + B1(a)	Digoxin, biotin	Litchfield et al. (1984)
Zymogen activation	A1 + B1(a)	Biotin	Blake et al. (1984)

of the method of detection of the label, together with the effect on the signal of antibody binding (Table 3; see also Nargessi and Landon, 1981). Until recently it had been assumed that a homogeneous assay using a radioactive label would be impossible. However, the recent reports of quenching of β emission by barium oxide producing a homogeneous immunoassay, and a homogeneous receptor binding assay based on radioluminescence (Tscharner and Bailey, 1983) appear to refute this assumption. Although some of these assays have found real application in the clinical laboratory, heterogeneous assays are still preferred by most assayists.

Present homogeneous assays suffer from four major problems:

(i) Many are dependent on the unique properties of a particular antibody or antigen and are therefore not applicable to all antibody–antigen reactions (Nargessi and Landon, 1981).

(ii) The detection limit of most of the labels is inferior to that of ^{125}I, in some cases by more than one order of magnitude.

(iii) Many of the homogeneous assays are interfered with by components of serum and other biological fluids (Ullman and Khanna, 1981).

Table 3. Classification of homogeneous interaction

A.   *Detection of label in antibody–antigen immunoassays*

   1. Spectrophotometry – enzyme label
   2. Fluorescence emission
   3. Fluorescence polarization
   4. Chemiluminescence
   5. Electron spin resonance
   6. Light scattering (nephelometry)
   7. Radioactivity

B.   *Change in signal induced by antibody–antigen interaction*

   1. Enhancement or reduction without a change in spectrum:

      (a) Alteration in ability of label to interact with another molecule (e.g. a substrate, an enzyme or antibody directed towards the label as opposed to the analyte)

      (b) Excited state quenching (direct or by energy transfer)

      (c) Enhancement of quantum yield

      (d) Change in light scattering or polarization

   2. Change in spectrum:

      (a) Excitation energy transfer

      (b) Rotational correlation in ESR

(iv) The apparatus and automation necessary for some of the homogeneous techniques is often expensive and complicated.

Chemiluminescent labels are easily detectable in the femtomole to atto-mole (10^{-15}–10^{-18} mol) range and potentially down to tipomoles (10^{-21} mol) (Campbell and Simpson, 1979; Campbell, 1983; Weeks *et al.*, 1983a,b; Campbell *et al.*, 1984). They are stable, apparently indefinitely on storage, and appear to be non-hazardous. Furthermore, they can be quantified simply within 1–10 s, and potentially within 0.1 s, a factor of considerable signi-ficance for large screening procedures involving thousands of samples. The aim of our work has been to apply the principle of chemiluminescence energy transfer to the development of a general homogeneous method for quantify-ing ligand–ligand interactions in living systems (Fig. 3). What then is chemiluminescence energy transfer?

3.   THE PHENOMENON OF ENERGY TRANSFER

Luminescence is the emission of light from atoms or molecules when returning to the ground state from electronically excited states. This defini-tion distinguishes it from incandescence where the energy for light emission arises from vibrational energy between atoms or molecules. Energy transfer from an electronically excited state to another molecule was predicted by Franck in 1922 and demonstrated in the vapour phase between excited

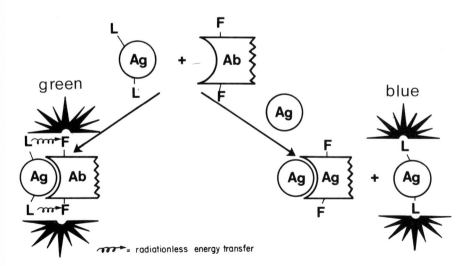

Fig. 3. The principle of chemiluminescent energy transfer immunoassay

mercury atoms and thallium by Cario and Franck in the following year (Cario and Franck, 1923).

Energy transfer in solution was first observed by Perrin and Choucroun (1929) as sensitized fluorescence from benzoflavine to rhodamine. Förster (1949), however, was only able to observe quenching of trypoflavine fluorescence by rhodamine. Nevertheless, the latter author established that this was non-radiative energy transfer, as opposed to the 'trivial' emission of a photon followed by reabsorption by the acceptor (Table 4), and that it required the donor and acceptor to be within 7 nm. A full mathematical treatment (Förster, 1948—translation available on request, 1959, 1966) led to the conclusion that the rate and efficiency of this type of energy transfer, dependent on dipole–dipole resonance, was related inversely to the sixth power of the distance between the excited donor and the acceptor. It was also critically dependent on the overlap integral between the emission spectrum of the donor and the excitation spectrum of the acceptor (Haugland *et al.*, 1969). It can thus be distinguished from radiative (trivial) and the other types of non-radiative energy transfer (Table 4).

The Förster equation predicting the efficiency of transfer between the lowest vibrational excited states (e.g. for chemiluminescence) by dipole–dipole resonance can be represented as follows:

$$\text{Efficiency, } E = d^{-6} / (d^{-6} + R_0^{-6}), \tag{1}$$

where d represents the distance in ångstroms between the centres of the donor and acceptor molecules. The value of the variable R_0 is given (also in ångstroms) by the equation

$$R_0 = (JK^2Q_0n^{-4})^{1/6} \times 9.7 \times 10^3. \tag{2}$$

Table 4. Energy transfer from an excited state donor to an acceptor molecule

---

A.   *Radiative (trivial)*: direct transfer of photon from donor to acceptor.

B.   *Non-radiative*: no direct transfer of a photon

    1. Exiton transfer: only applies to rigid materials (i.e. solids and glasses)

    2. Electron exchange (collisional): requires donor and acceptor orbitals overlap

    3. Electron transfer: requires donor and acceptor orbitals overlap

    4. Coulombic or resonance energy transfer (Förster): no orbital overlaps necessary, up to 10 nm, can be intra- or intermolecular

    5. Energy pooling: requires formation of an excimer or exiplex

---

See also Dexter (1953), Förster (1948, 1959, 1966), Lamola and Turro (1969)

This equation contains a number of spectroscopic variables: J is the spectral overlap integral (in cubic centimetres per mole) and is given by

$$J = \int F (\lambda) \, \epsilon \, (\lambda) \, \lambda^4 \, d\lambda \, / \int F(\lambda) \, d\lambda$$

(see Fig. 4); n is the refractive index of the medium between the donor and the acceptor; k_f is the rate constant for photon emission by the donor (i.e. the excited state arising from the chemiluminescent reaction); Q_0 is the quantum yield of the chemiluminescent energy donor in the absence of the acceptor. The rate of energy transfer (per second), k_T, is given by

$$k_T = CJd^{-6}, \tag{3}$$

where C is a constant given by

$$C = K^2 n^{-4} k_f \times 8.71 \times 10^{23}.$$

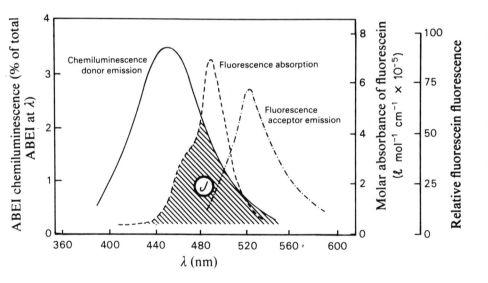

Fig. 4. J integral for ABEI chemiluminescence to fluorescein. The excitation (---) and emission (·—·—·) spectra of fluorescein were plotted from the data of Chen (1969), and confirmed by measurement using a Perkin-Elmer 204 A fluorescence spectrometer at pH 7.4 and 9. Chemiluminescence of ABEI (——) was measured at pH 9 using the dual photomultiplier luminometer, as described by Campbell and Patel (1983). Only one photomultiplier had an interference filter in front of it; the other was used as a reference to calculate ABEI light emission as a ratio of light at λ to total light recorded in the reference photomultiplier tube. [Reproduced from Campbell and Patel (1983) by permission of *The Biochemical Journal*.]

K^2 is the orientation factor for dipole–dipole interaction:

$$K^2 = \begin{cases} 0 & \text{when donor and acceptor are at right angles,} \\ 4 & \text{for perfect orientation,} \\ 2/3 & \text{for random orientation} \end{cases}$$

(Stryer, 1978).

The validity of Förster's mathematical treatment has been established using model fluorescent compounds (Latt et al., 1965; Stryer and Haugland, 1967; see Bowen, 1965, for a review). This type of energy transfer appears to play an important role in photosynthesis in prokaryote blue-green and eukaryote red algae (Tomita and Rabinowitch, 1962; Glazer, 1976). The chlorophyll of green plants absorbs light poorly in the 500–600 nm region, with the result that plants are unable to utilize the energy of one-third of the visible spectrum. Blue-green and red algae on the other hand contain protein micelles called phycobilosomes. These structures contain a group of phycocyanins which provide an energy transfer pathway to chlorophyll (French and Young, 1952; Brown et al., 1981). Interestingly the red luminous organ of the fish *Malacosteus niger* contains a blue–red fluorescent protein of similar spectral properties to a phycocyanin (A.K. Campbell, S.B. Matthews and P.J. Herring, unpublished). These proteins can be coupled to antibodies and haptens and may provide valuable fluors in cell sorting, immunocytochemistry and immunoassay (Vernon et al., 1982; Kronick and Grossman, 1983).

Non-radiative, resonance energy transfer has important application as a spectroscopic ruler (Stryer, 1978) and as a method for quantifying molecular movement (Stryer, 1982). Although uncertainty in the parameters of the Förster equation [(equation (1)] have limited the quantitative application of this phenomenon to biological systems it has been established that, to a first approximation, energy transfer is negligible once the donor and acceptor molecules are more than 5–10 nm apart (Stryer, 1978). This is important if energy transfer is to be used to establish a homogeneous immunoassay. The Stokes' radius of an IgG molecule of molecular weight 150 000 daltons is approximately 4 nm, and fluorescence energy transfer has established that the receptor sites on an antibody are 5.5. nm apart (Luedtke et al., 1980). Thus with between 4 and 12 molecules of fluor per antibody molecule at least one of them should be close enough and in the correct orientation to accept excitation energy from a donor on the antigen. Furthermore, a concentration of 1–10 mmol ℓ^{-1} of fluor is required before the donor and acceptor molecules are close enough in free solution to allow energy transfer to take place (Förster, 1948, 1959; Ward and Cormier, 1978). Yet under the conditions of an immunoassay the antibody concentration is usually in the range between 1 nmol l^{-1} and 1 pmol l^{-1}, or less. Thus an essential requirement of energy transfer immunoassay would be satisfied; it would only occur within the antibody–antigen complex and not between unassociated molecules.

Quenching of endogenous tryptophan fluorescence in an antibody by non-radiative energy transfer to its hapten, DNP-lysine, was first used to quantify antibody–antigen binding by Velick and co-workers (Velick, 1958; Velick et al., 1960). This method, however, was only applicable to pure antibodies and chromophoric haptens. Excitation of a fluorescent acceptor was established as a method for homogeneous immunoassay by Ullman and co-workers (Ullman et al., 1976; Khanna and Ullman, 1980; Ullman and Khanna, 1981; Table 2). Energy transfer is usually followed by quenching of the donor emission enabling homogeneous assays for a wide range of hapten and protein antigens to be established. A particular problem is the endogeneous fluorescence of serum and the usual limitations of detection of fluorescent labels. The analyte, therefore, must at present be at a concentration greater than 10 nmol l^{-1} in the sample. A further problem is the relative paucity of fluors with large extinction coefficients and high fluorescence quantum yields in aqueous solution. This is the reason for the popularity of fluorescein, rhodamine and umbelliferones (Chen, 1969). The new lucifer dyes and phycocyanin pigments may offer attractive alternatives in the future. Chemiluminescence energy transfer immunoassay should circumvent the problems of sensitivity encountered with simple fluorescence energy transfer.

4. THE SELECTION OF DONOR AND ACCEPTOR FOR CHEMILUMINESCENCE ENERGY TRANSFER

In order to select the most likely chemiluminescent donor and fluorescent acceptor for a homogeneous immunoassay, it is necessary first to re-examine the Förster equation [equation (1)]. We have no real control over parameters such as the refractive index n, K, and d. However, it is necessary to select a chemiluminescent substance with a high quantum yield which can be detected easily in the range 1–100 amol and which can be coupled to an antigen without significant loss of chemiluminescent or antigenic activity. Ideally the fluor should also have a high fluorescence quantum yield if a dual wavelength detection system is to be used (Fig. 2), and must have a good J integral (Fig. 4) with the excited product of the chemiluminescent reaction. Ideally, the Stokes' shift, i.e. the difference between the emission maximum of the donor and that of the acceptor, should also be large, e.g. blue–red, rather than blue–green.

Bioluminescent substances can be detected down to 10^{-20} mol (10 tmol), with very low chemical blanks, and could in theory provide valuable reagents for energy transfer immunoassays. The spectral emission maxima of most luminous marine organisms lies in the range 395–545 nm, the majority being within 450–490 nm, i.e. they emit blue light (O'Day and Fernandez, 1974; Fernandez, 1978; Herring, 1983). The excitation maximum of fluorescein is approximately 495 nm and thus the J integral with bioluminescent systems should be adequate. In contrast, terrestrial or freshwater luminous organisms usually emit at longer wavelengths, in the blue–green to yellow region, and could in theory undergo energy transfer with rhodamine (λ_{max} for excitation approx. 550 nm).

A particularly interesting feature of some marine bioluminescent spectra is that they are bimodal and may even change with time, as for example in Searsiid fish and in the amphipod *Parapronoë crustulum*. The railroad worm *Phrixothrix tiemanni* (Tiemann, 1970) and stomiatoid fish such as *Malacosteus niger* have light organs which emit different colours: red and green in the former and red and blue in the latter. It has, however, yet to be established whether any of these peculiar spectral features are the result of energy transfer.

In two groups of luminous organisms, certain bacteria and coelenterates, energy transfer has been demonstrated (Table 5). The luminous bacterium *Photobacterium phosphoreum* contains a blue fluorescent protein, lumazine, which binds to the luciferase–FMN complex and shifts the emission maximum from 490 nm *in vitro* to 472 nm *in vivo* (Gast and Lee, 1978; Lee and Koka, 1978; Koka and Lee, 1979; Visser and Lee, 1980, 1982; Small *et al.*, 1980; Lee, 1982; Vervoori *et al.*, 1983). One yellow strain (Y1) of this bacterium has even been reported (Ruby and Nealson, 1977), where the extracted luciferase–FMN complex still emits blue–green light *in vitro*. However, it has yet to be established whether this energy transfer occurs via dipole–dipole resonance or one of the other non-radiative mechanisms (Table 4), such as collisional or electron transfer, which require close contact between donor and acceptor.

A change in colour and an increase in quantum yield between three- and fivefold has been established between the luciferin-luciferase of *Renilla* and its green fluorescent protein (Ward and Cormier, 1976, 1978, 1979; Ward, 1979; Hart *et al.*, 1979). Although the process appears to be a Förster-type energy transfer, this process has yet to be fully established with coelenterates such as *Aequorea* and *Obelia* which contain photoproteins (Prendergast and Mann, 1978; Shimomura, 1979). It has even been suggested (Ward and Cormier, 1978) that radiative energy transfer may occur in these latter two organisms. However, energy transfer to the green fluorescent protein, or FMN, from aequorin has been observed whilst bound to a DEAE column (Morise *et al.*, 1974).

In addition to the question of feasibility of establishing such energy transfer within an antibody–antigen complex, bioluminescent reagents are not at present readily available in large quantities. Synthetic chemiluminescent compounds, however, can be prepared in gram quantities and several have been shown to undergo both intra- and intermolecular energy transfer (Table 5; see Ryzhikov, 1956; Rauhut, 1969; White *et al.*, 1974; Gunderman and Roeker, 1976; Faulkner, 1978; McCapra, 1978). Energy transfer forms an essential part of efficient light emission in the chemiluminescence of oxalyl

Table 5. Some proposed examples of chemiluminescence energy transfer

Proposed type of energy transfer (see Table 4)	Donor	Acceptor	References[†]
Radiative (A)	Aequorin	Green fluorescent protein	1, 20
Collisional (B2 or B3)	bacterial luciferase –FMN	Lumazine (blue)	2, 3
	bacterial luciferase –FMN	Yellow fluor	4
Electron transfer (B3)	oxalyl $Cl \rightarrow C_2O_4$	Anthracene	5
	oxalatester$\rightarrow C_2O_4$	Rubrene	6
	Diphenoyl peroxide$\rightarrow$ benzocoumarin	Rubrene	7, 8
	Dicyclohexyl peroxy-carbonate$\rightarrow$cyclo-hexanone	Rubrene	9
	Tetralin peroxide decomposition	Porphyrin	10
Intramolecular resonance (B4)	Phthalate	N-methyl acridone or anthracene	11, 12, 13, 14, 15
	aequorin	FMN	16
	aequorin-obelin	Green fluorescent protein	16, 17, 18, 19, 26
Intermolecular resonance (B4)	Phialidin	Green fluorescent protein	20
	Renilla oxyluciferin	Green fluorescent protein	1, 20, 21, 22
	Malacosteus oxyluciferin[‡]	Red fluor (?phycocyanin)	23, 24
Energy pooling (B5)	$^1O_2$	$^1O_2$	25

† *References*: 1, Ward *et al.* (1982); 2, Gast and Lee (1978); 3, Lee (1982); 4, Ruby and Nealson (1977); 5, Chandross (1963); 6, Rauhut (1969); 7 Koo and Schuster (1977); 8, Faulkner (1978); 9, Phillips *et al.* (1967); 10, Lundeen and Livingston (1965); 11, White and Roswell (1967, 1970); 12, Roberts and White (1970); 13, Ribi *et al.* (1972); 14, Roswell *et al.* (1970); 15, White *et al.* (1969); 16, Morise *et al.* (1974); 17, Morin and Hastings (1971); 18, Campbell and Hallett (1978); 19, Prendergast and Mann (1978); 20, Levine and Ward (1982); 21, Ward and Cormier (1976); 22, Ward (1979); 23, Herring (1983); 24, A. K. Campbell, S. B. Matthews and P. J. Herring (unpublished); 25, Gorman and Rodgers (1981); 26, Johnson *et al.* (1963)
‡ Not yet fully established; could be intramolecular.

chloride, oxalate esters, tetralin and peroxylates. However, these all appear to involve electron transfer to generate the excited state in the fluor via radical annihilation (Linschitz, 1961; Chandross, 1963; Hercules, 1969; Rauhut, 1969; Koo and Schuster, 1977; Faulkner, 1978). Similarly, electron transfer plays an essential part in electrochemically generated chemiluminescence (Sharifian and Park, 1982). Electron transfer requires close association, 0.2 nm, between donor and acceptor and is therefore unlikely to occur efficiently when the donor is some 1–5 nm from the acceptor, as it would be within an antibody–antigen complex.

The chemiluminescent donors chosen, therefore, for our initial experiments were aminobutylethylisoluminol (ABEI) and an acridinium ester (Fig. 5) which have adequate J integrals with fluorescein (Fig. 4) and have been coupled successfully to a range of antigens and antibodies for use in immunoassay (Schroeder et al., 1976a,b; Kohen et al., 1980; Pazzagli et al., 1981a,b; Kim et al., 1982; Patel et al., 1982; Weeks et al., 1983a; Campbell et al., 1984). Two other fluors were studied in addition to fluorescein (λ_{max} excitation 495 nm; emission 525 nm), namely, rhodamine (λ_{max} excitation 550 nm; emission 575 nm) and 4-chloro-7-nitrobenzo-2-oxa-1,3-diazole (NBD) (λ_{max} excitation 465 nm; emission 530 nm).

5. PREPARATION OF REAGENTS

For the initial experiments a hapten, cyclic AMP (molecular weight 329), and a protein antigen, rabbit IgG (molecular weight 150 000 daltons), were chosen to establish the principle of chemiluminescence energy transfer immunoassay. Succinyl cyclic AMP (scAMP) was covalently linked to ABEI by a mixed anhydride reaction using isobutyl chloroformate plus triethylamine (Campbell and Patel, 1983). ABEI–scAMP was purified by cellulose thin-layer chromatography and characterized by its ultraviolet absorption spectrum and immunological activity. ABEI was synthesized from 4-nitrophthalic acid with an overall yield of 2% by the method of Schroeder et al. (1978). It was converted to the isothiocyanate using thiophosgene (Patel et al., 1982), and then coupled to rabbit IgG at pH 9.5, producing up to 3 moles ABEI per mole of IgG, estimated spectrophotometrically or by chemiluminescence (Patel et al., 1983). Chemiluminescence of ABEI was assayed over the pH range 7.4–13 using microperoxidase + H_2O_2 as previously described (Patel et al., 1983; Campbell and Patel, 1983). Our home-built luminometer (EMI photomultiplier 9747 AM at between −940 and 1100V) was used, coupled to an Ecko M5060A scalar discriminator or home-built scalar interfaced to a LSI11 (RT11) computer. At pH 9 luminol generated 1.2×10^{19} luminescent cts mol^{-1}, ABEI or ABEI–IgG 2.1×10^{18} luminescent cts mol^{-1} and ABEI–scAMP 7.2×10^{18} luminescent cts mol^{-1}. The chemical background was 2000 luminescent counts in 10 s at pH 9. Although at pH 7.4 the luminescence of

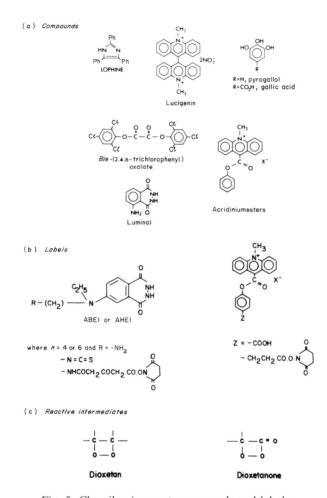

Fig. 5. Chemiluminescent compounds and labels

ABEI–scAMP was reduced approximately 10-fold so was the chemical blank.

Acridinium ester (McCapra and Richardson, 1964; McCapra et al., 1965) was coupled to rabbit IgG using an N-hydroxysuccinimide ester (Fig. 5; synthesized by Dr Iraj Beheshti). Acridinium ester was coupled to scAMP by the COOH group, but with a very low yield and was accompanied by over 90% hydrolysis of the ester to acridinium carboxylate, which is poorly chemiluminescent. Acridinium esters are highly luminescent at pH 13 in the presence of H_2O_2. However, at this pH, antibody–antigen complexes dissociate very rapidly. Hence, for the energy transfer experiments, microperoxidase plus H_2O_2 at pH 9 were used. Comparable problems with the acridinium esters arise at physiological pH because of the formation of pseudo-base (Weeks et al., 1983a).

The chemiluminescent labelled antigens were characterized by the following criteria: (i) chemical identity–ultraviolet spectra, fluorescence spectra, chemiluminescence; (ii) luminescent counts per mole at pH 7.4, 9 and 13; (iii) stability at -20 °C (more than 12 months), 20 °C, 37 °C at pH 7.4, 9 and 13; (iv) immunological activity by competition with ^{3}H or ^{125}I label and using chemiluminescence (K_D approximately the same as radioactive counterpart); (v) kinetics unaffected by antigen coupling or binding to antibody; (vi) quantum yield unaffected by antibody binding (in contrast to the reports of Schroeder et al., 1976b, and Pazzagli et al., 1981a).

Fluorescein (4–12 mol mol^{-1}) and rhodamine (6–8 mol mol^{-1}) were coupled to antibodies using their isothiocyanate derivatives at pH 9.5; NBD-Cl was coupled directly at pH 8 (3.0–6.2 mol mol^{-1}).

6. DEMONSTRATION OF CHEMILUMINESCENCE ENERGY TRANSFER

Using a dual wavelength photomultiplier luminometer to measure the functional chemiluminescence at a particular wavelength (Balzer filters, 7 nm half bandwidth), a reduction of light emission at 460 and 487 nm and an increase at 525 and 555 nm was observed when ABEI–rabbit IgG bound to its fluorescein-labelled antibody (Fig. 6, Patel et al., 1983). No such spectral shifts were seen when equivalent amounts of ABEI–rabbit IgG bound to unlabelled sheep anti-rabbit IgG, nor when ABEI–rabbit IgG was incubated with fluorescein-labelled non-immune sheep IgG. This non-radiative chemiluminescence energy transfer could be detected over the pH range 7.4–9, but not at pH 13 where rapid antibody–antigen dissociation occurs.

However, no energy transfer could be detected when rhodamine or NBD were used as acceptors for ABEI chemiluminescence, nor when using acridinium esters with fluorescein as acceptor (Fig. 7). Rhodamine has a poor J integral with ABEI chemiluminescence and NBD fluorescence may have been susceptible to the hydrophobicity within the antibody, or the pH and the H$_2$O$_2$ required for triggering ABEI chemiluminescence. Acridinium ester chemiluminescence results in the formation of an excited state N-methyl acridone (McCapra et al., 1965; Rauhut et al., 1965a,b) detached from the ester moiety coupled to the antigen or antibody (Weeks et al., 1983a). Since there is a 10-fold lower chemical background, acridinium esters offer advantages over ABEI as non-isotopic labels in heterogeneous immunoassays. However, until a method can be developed to retain them bound within the antibody–antigen complex, energy transfer immunoassay either by quenching or by excitation of the acceptor may be difficult to achieve.

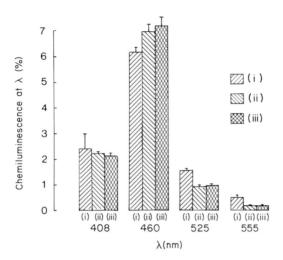

Fig. 6. Chemiluminescence of ABEI rabbit IgG + fluorescein–antibody at four wavelengths. Fifty microlitres $(1.67 \times 10^{-13}$ mol) of chemiluminescence-labelled rabbit IgG (0.2 moles ABEI per mole of IgG) in 50 mM phosphate buffer, pH 7.4, containing 0.01% bovine serum albumin, was incubated overnight at 4 °C with (i) 50 µl $(2 \times 10^{-10}$ mol) of fluorescein-labelled sheep anti-rabbit IgG (4 mol fluorescein per mole of IgG) or (ii) 50 µl $(3 \times 10^{-10}$ mol) of fluorescein-labelled sheep anti-human albumin IgG (3 moles fluorescein per mole of IgG) or (iii) 50 µl $(2 \times 10^{-10}$ mol) of unlabelled sheep anti-rabbit IgG. Under these conditions the fluorescent-labelled (i) and the unlabelled (iii) sheep anti-rabbit IgG bound more than 95% of chemiluminescent-labelled rabbit IgG, whereas the binding to non-specific fluorescent IgG (ii) was less than 5%, measured by antibody dilution curves. Chemiluminescence was activated with H_2O_2 + microperoxidase, and detected at various wavelengths using the specially constructed dual photomultiplier luminometer. One photomultiplier tube was used as a reference, measuring total light from the reaction, while the second photomultiplier tube measured the light at a particular wavelength using metal film interference filters (Balzers Ltd, Berkhamstead, Herts, UK, Type B40 of narrow half bandwidth (7 nm)]. Chemiluminescence from blank tubes containing anti-IgG and buffer instead of ABEI-rabbit IgG was deducted. The percentage of chemiluminescence at each wavelength was calculated relative to the total chemiluminescence measured in the reference photomultiplier tube. Each value represents the mean ± S.D. of three determinations at each wavelength. No corrections for the geometry of the apparatus, the transmission of the filters, or the spectral response of the photomultiplier tubes were made

7. OPTIMIZATION OF ENERGY TRANSFER

In order to establish the optimum conditions for a homogeneous immunoassay based on a chemiluminescence energy transfer, ABEI was compared with an acridinium ester chemiluminescent label (Fig. 5). The use of fluorescein as the energy transfer acceptor was compared with rhodamine and NBD (Fig.

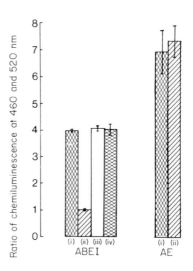

Fig. 7. Effect of different chemiluminescent labels and fluors on energy transfer. Experimental conditions as Fig. 6. (i) ▨ unlabelled sheep anti-rabbit Ig; (ii) ▨ fluorescein sheep anti-rabbit IgG; (iii) ☐ NBD sheep anti-rabbit IgG; (iv) ▨ rhodamine sheep anti-rabbit IgG. ABEI, ABEI-labelled rabbit IgG; AE, acridinium ester-labelled rabbit IgG

7). Chemiluminescence was measured at two wavelengths simultaneously (460 and 525 nm for fluorescein, NBD and rhodamine, and also at 460 and 572 nm for rhodamine) using the dual wavelength luminometer (Fig. 2). The ratio of chemiluminescence at both wavelengths was estimated after subtraction of the chemical blank (H_2O_2 + microperoxidase only). This improved the standard deviation in the ratios some five- to 10-fold compared with measurement at a single wavelength, particularly since it reduced errors due to irreproducible mixing between samples. ABEI was selected as the chemiluminescent donor and fluorescein as the acceptor, since no significant energy transfer could be detected with the other pairs (as discussed above).

Energy transfer was detected within the antibody–antigen complex using a range of haptens and protein antigens of molecular weights between 312 and 150 000 daltons; Fig. 8). The chemiluminescence ratio at 460 nm (blue) to 525 nm (green) decreased by approximately 50–70% when more than 95% of the labelled antigen was bound to fluorescein-labelled antibody. The reason for the smaller change in ratios obtained with ABEI–scGMP is not known.

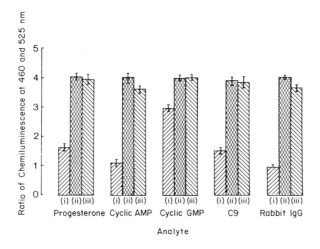

Fig. 8. Chemiluminescence energy transfer with different analytes. Chemiluminescent labelled antigens were synthesized as described, and incubated with fluorescein-labelled or unlabelled antibodies (IgG, binding > 95% of antigen), or fluorescein-labelled non-immune IgG for 2 h at room temperature (approx. 20 °C) in 100 μl of 100 mM sodium barbitone, pH 9. Chemiluminescence was activated by adding 100 μl of 4 μM microperoxidase in 100 mM barbitone buffer, pH 9, containing 0.01 g of bovine serum albumin per 100 ml, followed by 20 μl of 175 mM H_2O_2 in water. Light emission was monitored at 460 nm and 525 nm simultaneously and the ratio was calculated. Results represent the mean ± S.D. of three observations. (i) ▨ fluorescein-labelled immune IgG; (ii) ▨ unlabelled immune IgG; (iii) ▨ fluorescein-labelled non-immune IgG

8. HOMOGENEOUS CHEMILUMINESCENCE ENERGY TRANSFER IMMUNOASSAY

In order to establish the concentration of fluorescein-labelled antibody necessary for a homogeneous immunoassay an antibody dilution curve was carried out over the range 1 : 500 to 1 : 5 (c. 14–1400 μg IgG ml^{-1}). The ratio of luminescence at 460 nm to that at 525 nm decreased from 4.0 to 1.3 for ABEI–scAMP (Fig. 9), and similarly for rabbit IgG, complement component C9, progesterone and adenosine (ABEI–laevulinyl adenosine) (Fig. 8). Unlabelled anti-analyte IgG produced no shift towards the green. Fluorescein-labelled non-immune IgG produced only a small shift at 1 : 5 dilution where some energy transfer may have occurred with free ABEI–antigen, or where there was some non-specific binding.

Using a fluorescein IgG dilution equivalent to approximately 50% binding, dose–response curves for rabbit IgG (Fig. 10a) (17 fmol–170 pmol), comple-

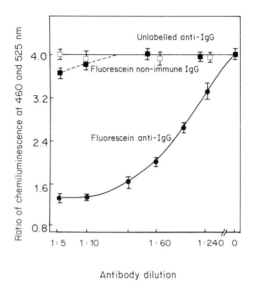

Antibody dilution

Fig. 9. Antibody dilution curve. ABEI –scAMP (50 μl of 10 nM) was incubated with 25 μl of 50 mM sodium phosphate, pH 7.4, containing 0.1 g of human IgG per 100 ml and 25 μl of fluorescein-labelled anti-(cyclic AMP) IgG (●–●), 25 μl of unlabelled anti-(cyclic AMP) IgG (□–□), or 25 μl of fluorescein-labelled non-immune IgG (■–■), for 2 h at room temperature. The concentration of IgG in all the undiluted solutions was 7 mg ml^{-1}; dilutions are as shown. Chemiluminescence was initiated by adding 100 μl of 5 μM microperoxidase in 100 mM sodium barbitone, pH 9, containing 10 mg of bovine serum albumin per 100 ml, followed by 20 μl of 0.175 M H$_2$O$_2$. Light emission at 460 and 525 nm was measured simultaneously. Results represent the mean ± S.D. for three determinations [Reproduced from Campbell and Patel (1983) by permission of *The Biochemical Journal*.]

ment component C9 (0.1–1000 ng), cyclic AMP (25 fmol–2.5 pmol), and progesterone (0.88 pmol–8.8 nmol) (Campbell and Patel, 1983; Patel and Campbell, 1983) and adenosine (25 pmol–25 nmol) were established. The dose–response curves were usually established at pH 7.4 and the ABEI chemiluminescence triggered at pH 9. If the ABEI was also assayed at pH 7.4 there was a reduction of some 10-fold in sensitivity (Campbell and Patel, 1983) because of the need for a 10-fold increase in the concentration of fluorescein IgG and ABEI–scAMP.

The homogeneous assays could be used to measure cyclic AMP extracted from pigeon erythrocytes and IgG in samples of rabbit serum. These measurements correlated well with results by conventional heterogeneous radioimmunoassay (cyclic AMP: $y = 1.18x + 0.68$, $r = 0.91$, $n = 17$; IgG: $y = 1.01x - 0.23$, $r = 0.96$, $n = 13$, see Fig. 10b).

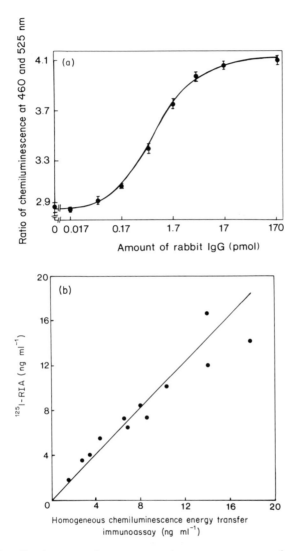

Fig. 10. (a) Chemiluminescence immunoassay dose–response curve for rabbit IgG. Standard rabbit IgG solutions (25 μl, $6.7 \times 10^{-10} - 6.7 \times 10^{-6}$ M) in 50 mM phosphate buffer, pH 7.4, containing 0.01% bovine serum albumin were incubated with 50 μl chemiluminescent-labelled rabbit IgG (3.33×10^{-9} M) and 25 μl of fluorescein-labelled sheep anti-rabbit IgG (1×10^{-7} M; binds 50% label) overnight at 4 °C. The amount of chemiluminescent label bound to the fluorescent antibody was assessed by measuring the chemiluminescence at the two wavelengths, 460 and 525 nm, simultaneously using two interference filters and measuring the ratio of luminescence at the two wavelengths. Each point represents the mean ± S.D. of three determinations. [Reproduced from Patel *et al.* (1983) by permission of Academic Press.] (b) Correlation between ^{125}I radioimmunoassay and homogeneous assay for IgG in rabbit serum

A problem with many homogeneous immunoassays is interference with label detection by serum (Ullman and Khanna, 1981). High serum concentrations (>10%) do decrease ABEI chemiluminescence (Fig. 11). This effect could be due to protein quenching the excited state, or to interference with the catalytic reaction. The decrease was greater at pH 13 than at pH 9, possibly because of denaturation and precipitation of serum proteins, though changes in turbidity and light scattering are much less of a problem with chemiluminescence than fluorescence. A major advantage of the ratio method of detecting energy transfer (Fig. 2) is that it self-compensates for any effect of biological samples on the kinetics and quantum yield of the chemiluminescence.

A further application of this homogeneous immunoassay technique is that the association and dissociation of ABEI-labelled antigens with their respective fluorescein-labelled antibodies can also be quantified (Fig. 12) over the pH range 7–9 and the temperature range 0–37 °C. This development now makes ligand binding to low affinity, fast dissociating antibodies and other binding proteins accessible to quantitative study.

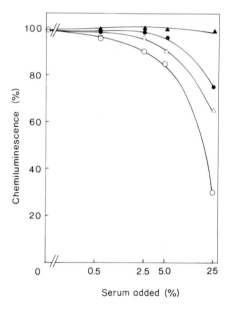

Fig. 11. Effect of serum on ABEI chemiluminescence. To 50 μl of 10 nM ABEI in phosphate buffer, pH 7.4, containing 0.01% BSA was added 50 μl of varying dilutions of either rabbit serum (△, ▲) or human serum (○, ●). The chemiluminescence of the ABEI was then measured using the microperoxidase–H_2O_2 assay at pH 9.0 (▲, ●) or at pH 13.0 (△, ○). The percentage inhibition of the chemiluminescence without any serum added is shown

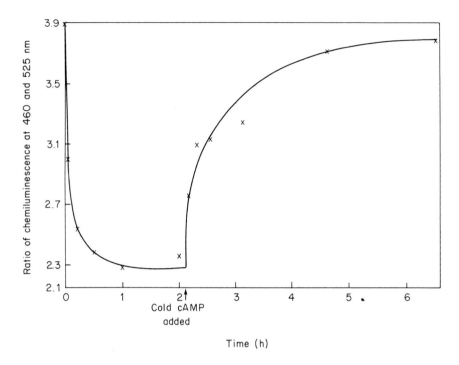

Fig. 12. Association and dissociation of antibody–antigen complex by energy transfer. The binding and dissociation of ABEI–succinyl-cAMP to fluorescent-labelled anti-bodies was detected in an homogeneous assay using chemiluminescence energy transfer. An aliquot (1.3 ml) of ABEI–succinyl-cAMP (1×10^{-8} M) in phosphate buffer containing 0.1% human IgG, pH 7.4, was added to 650 μl of the appropriate dilution of fluorescent-labelled anti-cAMP IgG and mixed. Aliquots (75 μl) were removed at timed intervals and mixed with 25 μl of buffer and the ratio of the chemiluminescence at 460 nm and 525 nm measured as described previously. After 2 h, 500 μl of 1×10^{-3} M cyclic AMP was added to 1 ml of the mixture and 100 μl aliquots were removed at timed intervals and the chemiluminescence was measured as above. The ratio of the chemiluminescence counts at 460 nm and 525 nm was then plotted against time. Each point represents the mean of two determinations. [Reproduced from Patel *et al.* (1983) by permission of Academic Press.]

9. APPLICATIONS IN CELL BIOLOGY

Conventionally chemical analysis of tissues involves the measurement of extracts of thousands, if not millions of cells. These studies have two major limitations. Firstly, many chemical events occur only while the cell remains intact. Secondly, they cannot take into account heterogeneity within the cell population. It has been proposed that many types of cell activation, including cell movement, muscle contraction, cell division, secretion and the reversal of the direction of intermediary metabolism, are 'threshold' phenomena (Campbell, 1983). It has further been proposed that several of these are triggered by intracellular Ca^{2+} and modified by cyclic nucleotides. A crucial test of this hypothesis is the measurement of second messengers and cell activation in single, intact cells. Several pathological phenomena, for example the effect of the membrane attack complex of complement, may also exhibit thresholds at the level of individual cells.

We have developed three methods for incorporating luminescent indicators into functional cells: (i) cell 'ghosts' (Campbell and Dormer, 1978); (ii) cell hybridization using erythrocyte 'ghosts' and fusion induced by Sendai virus (Hallett and Campbell, 1982b); (iii) release of material from micropinocytotic vesicles into the cell cytoplasm (Hallett and Campbell, 1983).

Three problems have been encountered with ABEI–scAMP. Firstly, phosphodiesterase degrades the cAMP moiety both in the test tube and within the cell. Although this destruction can be inhibited by 3-isobutyl-methylxanthine (IBMX), more than 50% of the immunological activity can be lost within a few minutes. Secondly, H_2O_2 is necessary for ABEI chemiluminescence. This substance, together with oxygen radicals, can be very toxic to cells and appears to cross the cell membrane very slowly. Concentrations as high as 0.1–1 mM outside the cell are necessary to stimulate the chemiluminescence of ABEI within. Thirdly, ABEI chemiluminescence is pH sensitive, and inefficient at physiological values. Our present studies are aimed at using bioluminescent systems which utilize O_2 directly, to circumvent these problems.

10. CONCLUSIONS AND FUTURE PROSPECTS

Non-radiative chemiluminescence energy transfer occurs through dipole–dipole resonance between the excited reaction product as donor and an acceptor. Our results demonstrate, using ABEI as the donor and fluorescein as the acceptor, that this phenomenon can occur within an antibody–antigen complex. This phenomenon can be used to quantify antibody–antigen reactions without the need of a separation step. The resulting homogeneous immunoassays appear to be comparable with their radioactive counterparts, and potentially more sensitive—particularly if the reaction is carried out in very small volumes (e.g. 0.1–1 μl). Furthermore, they appear considerably more sensitive than other reported homogeneous immunoassays (Table 2), and are less susceptible to interference from substances in biological samples—mainly due to the fact that measurements are carried out at two wavelengths simultaneously (Fig. 2). It is now necessary to: (i) establish the clinical validity of this homogeneous immunoassay principle; :(ii) improve the detection of the chemiluminescent label and the J integral (Fig. 4) by selecting new donor–acceptor pairs; and (iii) use this method to study chemical changes in single and intact cells.

The advancement of medical science is dependent not simply on the development of new techniques, but critically on conceptual advances in our understanding of pathogenic mechanisms. This framework then provides new approaches to the diagnosis and treatment of disease. The establishment of homogeneous methods for studying ligand–ligand interactions in living systems provides exciting opportunities for the chemical characterization of individual human cells. The two major limitations of the conventional biochemical approach can thus be circumvented, enabling a new approach to cell activation and injury to be developed.

ACKNOWLEDGEMENTS

We thank the Medical Research Council, the Science and Engineering Research Council, the Arthritis and Rheumatism Council and the Department of Health and Social Security for financial support. We thank the Director and staff of the Marine Biological Association Laboratory, Plymouth, and Dr Peter J. Herring and the crew of RRS *Discovery* for much help. We also thank Malcolm E. T. Ryall for construction of luminometers. Dr Michael M. Morton and Christopher J. Davies for help with the synthesis of ABEI, Dr Brian Joyce for the kind gift of progesterone antisera, Dr A. Newby for adenosine antisera, Dr B. Paul Morgan for C9 antisera and Dr K. Siddle for cyclic nucleotide antisera. Finally we thank Iraj Beheshti for the acridinium ester label and Professor McCapra for many helpful discussions.

REFERENCES

Arquilla, E. R. and Stavitsky, A. M. (1956). The production and identification of antibodies to insulin and their use in assaying insulin. *J. Clin. Invest.* **35**, 458–466.

Ashley, C. C. and Campbell, A. K. (1979). *The Detection and Measurement of Free Ca^{2+} in Cells*. Elsevier–North Holland, Amsterdam.

Berson, S. A. and Yalow, R. S. (1959). Quantitative aspects of the reaction between insulin and insulin-binding antibody. *J. Clin. Invest.* **38**, 1996–2016.

Blake, D. A., Skarstedt, M. T., Schultz, J. L. and Wilson, D. P. (1984). Zymogen activation. A new system for homogeneous ligand-binding assay. *Clin. Chem.* **30**, 1452–1456.

Bowen, E. J. (1965). Electronic energy transfer processes. In *Energy Transfer in Radiation Processes* (G. O. Phillips, ed.), Elsevier, Amsterdam, pp. 6–14.

Brown, S. B., Holroyd, A., Troxler, R. F. and Offner, G. D. (1981). Bile pigment synthesis in plants: incorporation of haem into phycocyanobilin and phycobiliproteins in *Cyanidium caldarium*. *Biochem. J.* **194**, 137–147.

Burd, J. F. (1981). The homogeneous substrate-labelled fluorescent immunoassay. *Meth. Enzymol.* **74 C**, 79–87.

Campbell, A. K. (1974). Extraction, partial purification and properties of obelin, the Ca^{2+}-activated photoprotein from the hydroid *Obelia geniculata*. *Biochem. J.* **143**, 411–418.

Campbell, A. K. (1983). *Intracellular Calcium: Its Universal Role as Regulator*, John Wiley, Chichester.

Campbell, A. K. and Dormer, R. L. (1978). Inhibition by calcium of cyclic AMP formation in sealed pigeon erythrocyte 'ghosts': a study using the photoprotein obelin. *Biochem. J.* **176**, 53–66.

Campbell, A. K. and Hallett, M. B. (1978). Luminescence in cells and vesicles isolated from the hydroid *Obelia geniculata*. *J. Physiol., Lond.* **287**, 4–5P.

Campbell, A. K. and Patel, A. (1983). A homogeneous immunoassay for cyclic nucleotides based on chemiluminescence energy transfer. *Biochem. J.* **216**, 185–194.

Campbell, A. K. and Simpson, J. S. A. (1979). Chemi- and bioluminescence as an analytical tool in biology. *Tech. Life Sci. (Metabolic Res.)* **B213**, 1–56.

Campbell, A. K., Lea, T. J. and Ashley, C. C. (1979). In *Detection and Measurement of Free Ca²⁺ in Cells.* (C. C. Ashley and A. K. Campbell, eds), Elsevier–North Holland, Amsterdam, pp. 13–72.

Campbell, A. K., Davies, C. J., Hart, R., McCapra, F., Patel, A., Richardson, A., Ryall, M. E. T., Simpson, J. S. A. and Woodhead, J. S. (1980). Chemiluminescent labels in immunoassay. *J. Physiol., Lond.* **306**, 4–5P.

Campbell, A. M., Holt, M. and Patel, A. (1984). Chemiluminescence as an analytical tool in medical biochemistry. *Recent Adv. Clin. Chem.* **3**, in press.

Cario, G. and Franck, J. (1923). [Sensitized fluorescence of gases.] *Z. Phys.* **17**, 202–212 (in German).

Chandross, E. A. (1963). A new chemiluminescent system. *Tetrahedron Lett.* 761–765.

Chen, R. F. (1969). Fluorescent protein–dye conjugates. II. Gamma globulin conjugated with various dyes. *Archs. Biochem. Biophys.* **133**, 263–276.

Crowl, C. P., Gibbons, I. and Schneider, R. S. (1980). In *Immunoassays: Clinical Laboratory Techniques for the 1980s.* (R.N. Nakamura, R. W. Dito and E. S. Tucker, eds), Alan R. Liss, Inc. New York, pp. 89–126.

Dandliker, W. B. and Feigen, G. (1961). Quantification of the antigen–antibody reaction by the polarization of fluorescence. *Biochem. Biophys. Res. Commun.* **5**, 299.

Dexter, D. L. (1953). A theory of sensitised luminescence in solids. *J. Phys. Chem.* **21**, 836–850.

Faulkner, L. R. (1978). Chemiluminescence from electron-transfer processes. *Meth. Enzymol.* **57**, 494–526.

Fernandez, H. R. C. (1978). Visual pigments of bioluminescent and non-bioluminescent deep-sea fishes. *Vision Res.* **19**, 589–592.

Förster, T. (1948). Zwischenmoleculare Energiewanderung und Fluoreszenz. *Annln. Phys.* **2**, 55–75.

Förster, T. (1949). Experiments on intermolecular transition of electron excitation energy. *Z. Electrochemie* **53**, 93–99.

Förster, T. (1959). Transfer mechanisms of electronic excitation. *Disc. Faraday Soc.* **27**, 7–17.

Förster, T. (1966). Delocalised excitation and excitation transfer. In *Modern Quantum Chemistry*, Vol. IIIB (D. Sinanoglu, ed.), Academic Press, New York, pp. 93–137.

Franck, J. (1922). Einige aus der Theorie von Klein und Rosseland zu ziehende Folgerungen über Fluoreszenz, photochemische Prozesse und die Elektronenemission glühender Körper. *Z. Phys.* **9**, 259–260.

French, C. S. and Young, V. K. (1952). The fluorescence spectra of red algae and the transfer of energy from phycoerythrin to phycocyanin and chlorophyll. *J. Gen. Physiol.* **35**, 873–890.

Gast, R. and Lee, J. (1978). Isolation of the *in vivo* emitter in bacterial bioluminescence. *Proc. Natn. Acad. Sci. U.S.A.* **75**, 833–837.

Gibbons, I., Skold C., Rowley, G. L. and Ullman, E. F. (1980). Homogeneous enzyme immunoassay for proteins employing β-galactosidase. *Analyt. Biochem.* **102**, 167–170.

Glazer, A. N. (1976). Phycocyanins: structure and function. *Photochem. Photobiol. Rev.* **1**, 71–115.

Gorman, A. A. and Rodgers, M. A. S. (1981). Singlet molecular oxygen. *Q. Rev. Chem. Soc. (Chem. Soc. Rev.)* **10**, 205–231.

Gunderman, K. D. and Roeker, K. D. (1976) Konstitution und chemilumineszenz. VII. Chemilumineszierender Paracyclophane: II. Intramolekular sensibilisierte Chemilumineszenz. *Justis Liebigs Annln Chem.* **1**, 140–152.

Hallett, M. B. and Campbell, A. K. (1982a). Applications of coelenterate photoproteins. In *Clinical and Biochemical Luminescence* (J. J. Kricka and T. N. Carter, eds), Marcel Dekker, New York, pp. 89–113.

Hallett, M. B. and Campbell, A. K. (1982b). Measurement of changes in cytoplasmic free Ca^{2+} in fused cell hybrids. *Nature, Lond.* **295**, 155–158.

Hallett, M. B. and Campbell, A. K. (1983). Direct measurement of intracellular free Ca^{2+} in rat peritoneal macrophages: correlation with oxygen radical production. *Immunology* **50**, 487–495.

Hart, R. C., Matthews, J. C., Hori, K. and Cormier, M. J. (1979). *Renilla reniformis* bioluminescence: luciferase-catalyzed production of non-radiating excited states from luciferin analogues and elucidation of the excited state species involved in energy transfer to *Renilla* green fluorescent protein. *Biochemistry* **18**, 2204–2210.

Haugland, R. P., Yguerabide, J. and Stryer, L. (1969). Dependence of the kinetics of singlet–singlet energy transfer on spectral overlap. *Proc. Natn. Acad. Sci. U.S.A.* **63**, 23–30.

Hercules, D. M. (1969). Chemiluminescence from electron-transfer reactions. *Acc. Chem. Res.* **2**, 301–307.

Herring, P.J. (1983). The spectral characteristics of luminous marine organisms. *Proc. R. Soc. B* **220**, 183–217.

Johnson, F. H., Shimomura, O., Saiga, L. C., Gershman, G. T., Reynolds, G. T. and Waters, J. R. (1963). Quantum efficiency of *Cypridina* luminescence. *J. Cell. Comp. Physiol.* **60**, 85–104.

Khanna, P.J. and Ullman, E.F. (1980). 4′,5′-Dimethyl-6-carboxyfluorescein: a novel dipole–dipole coupled fluorescence energy transfer acceptor useful for fluorescence immunoassay. *Analyt. Biochem.* **108**, 156–161.

Kim, J. B., Barnard, G. J., Collins, W. P., Kohen, F., Lindner, H. R. and Eshhar, Z. (1982). Measurement of plasma estradiol-17β by solid-phase chemiluminescence immunoassay. *Clin. Chem.* **28**, 1120–1124.

Kohen, F., Pazzagli, M., Kim, J. B., Lindner, H. R. and Boguslaski, R. C. (1979). An assay procedure for plasma progesterone based on antibody-enhanced chemiluminescence. *FEBS Lett.* **104**, 201–205.

Kohen, F., Kim, J. B., Barnard, G. and Lindner, H. R. (1980). An immunoassay for urinary esteriol-16α-glucuronide based on antibody-enhanced chemiluminescence. *Steroids* **36**, 405–420.

Koka, P. and Lee, J. (1979). Separation and structure of the prosthetic group of the blue fluorescence protein from the bioluminescent bacterium *Photobacterium phosphoreum*. *Proc. Natn. Acad. Sci. U.S.A.* **76**, 3068–3072.

Koo, J.-Y. and Schuster, G. B. (1977). Chemically initiated electron exchange luminescence. A new chemiluminescent reaction path for organic peroxides. *J. Am. Chem. Soc.* **99**, 6107–6109.

Kronick, M. N. and Grossman, P. D. (1983). Immunoassay techniques with fluorescent phycobiliprotein conjugates. *Clin. Chem.* **29**, 1582–1586.

Lamola, A. A. and Turro, N. J. (1969). *Energy Transfer and Organic Photochemistry, Techniques of Organic Chemistry*, Vol. 14, Interscience, New York.

Latt, S. A., Cheung, H. T. and Blout, E. R. (1965). Energy transfer. A system with relatively fixed donor–acceptor separation. *J. Am. Chem. Soc.* **87**, 995–1003.

Lee, J. (1982). Sensitization by lumazine proteins of the bioluminescence emission from the reaction of bacterial luciferases. *Photochem. Photobiol.* **36**, 689–697.

Lee, J. and Koka, P. (1978). Purification of a blue-fluorescent protein from the bioluminescent bacterium *Photobacterium phosphoreum*. *Meth. Enzymol.* **57**, 226–234.

Leute, R. K., Ullman, E. F., Goldstein, A. and Herzenberg, L. H. (1972). Spin immunoassay technique for determination of morphine. *Nature New Biol.* **236**, 93–94.

Levine, L. D. and Ward, W. W. (1982). Isolation and characterisation of a photoprotein 'phialidin', and a spectrally unique green-fluorescent protein from the bioluminescent jellyfish *Phialidium gregarium*. *Comp. Biochem. Physiol.* **72**, 77–85.

Lim, C. S., Miller, J. N. and Bridges, J. W. (1980). Energy transfer immunoassay: a study of the experimental parameters in an assay for human serum albumin. *Analyt. Biochem.* **108**, 176–184.

Linschitz, H. (1961). Light emission by chemical reactions. In *Light and Life* (W. D. McElroy and B. Glass, eds) Johns Hopkins University Press, Baltimore, Md, pp. 173–183.

Litchfield, W. J., Freytag, J. W. and Adamich, M. (1984). Highly sensitive immunoassays based on the use of liposomes without complement. *Clin. Chem.* **30**, 1441–1445.

Luedtke, R., Owen, C. S. and Karwin, F. (1980). Proximity of antibody binding sites studied by fluorescence energy transfer. *Biochemistry* **19**, 1182–1192.

Lundeen, G. and Livingston, R. (1965). Chemiluminescence of hydrocarbon oxidation. *Photochem. Photobiol.* **4**, 1085.

McCapra, F. (1978). The chemistry of bioluminescence. In *Bioluminescence in Action* (P.J. Herring, ed.), Academic Press, London, pp. 49–73.

McCapra, F. and Richardson, D. G. (1964). Mechanism of chemiluminescence. New chemiluminescent reaction. *Tetrahedron Lett.* **43**, 3167–3172.

McCapra, F., Richardson, D. G. and Chang, Y. C. (1965). Chemiluminescence involving peroxide decompositions. *Photochem. Photobiol.* **4**, 1111–1121.

Morin, J. G. (1974). Coelenterate bioluminescence. In *Coelenterate Biology: Reviews and New Perspectives* (L. Muscatine and H. M. Lenhoff, eds), Academic Press, New York, pp. 397–438.

Morin, J. G. and Hastings, J. W. (1971). Energy transfer in a bioluminescent system. *J. Cell. Physiol.* **77**, 313–318.

Morise, H., Shimomura, O., Johnson, F. H. and Winant, J. (1974). Intermolecular energy transfer in the bioluminescent system of *Aequorea*. *Biochemistry* **13**, 2656–2662.

Nargessi, R. D. and Landon, J. (1981). Indirect quenching fluoroimmunoassay. *Meth. Enzymol.* **74C**, 60–79.

O'Day, W. T. and Fernandez, H. R. (1974). *Aristostomias scintillans* (Malacosteidae): a deep sea fish with visual pigments apparently adapted to its own bioluminescence. *Vision Res.* **14**, 545–560.

Patel, A. and Campbell, A. K. (1983). Homogeneous immunoassay based on chemiluminescence energy transfer. *Clin. Chem.* **29**, 1604–1608.

Patel, A., Morton, M. S., Woodhead, J. S., Ryall, M.E.T., McCapra, F. and Campbell, A. K. (1982). A new chemiluminescent label for use in immunoassay. *Biochem. Soc. Trans.* **10**, 224–225.

Patel, A., Davies, C. J., Campbell, A. K. and McCapra, F. (1983). Chemiluminescence energy transfer: a new technique applicable to the study of ligand–ligand interactions in living systems. *Analyt. Biochem.* **129**. 162–169.

Pazzagli, M., Kim, J. B., Messeri, G., Martinazzo, G., Kohen, F., Franceschetti, F., Moneti, G., Saherno, R., Tomassi, A. and Serio, M. (1981a). Evaluation of different progesterone–isoluminol conjugates for chemiluminescence immunoassay. *Clin. Chim. Acta* **115**, 277–286.

Pazzagli, M., Kim, J. B., Messeri, G., Martinazzo, G., Kohen, F., Franceschetti, F., Tomassi, A., Salerno, R. and Serio, M. (1981b). Luminescent immunoassay (LIA) for progesterone in a heterogeneous system. *Clin. Chim. Acta* **115**, 287–296.

Pazzagli, M., Bolleli, G. F., Messeri, G., Martinazzo, G., Tommasi, A., Salerno, R. and Serio, M. (1982). In *Luminescent Assays: Perspectives in Endocrinology and Clinical Chemistry* (M. Serio and M. Pazzagli, eds), Raven Press, New York, pp. 191–200.

Perrin, J. and Choucroun, N. (1929). Fluorescence sensitized in a liquid medium (transfer of activation by molecular induction). *C. R. hebd. Séanc. Acad. Sci., Paris* **189**, 1213–1216.

Philips, D., Anissimov, V., Karpukhin, O. and Shliupintokh, V. (1967). Energy transfer from chemiluminescent species in polymers. *Nature, Lond.* **215**, 1163–1165.

Prendergast, F. G. and Mann, K. G. (1978). Chemical and physical properties of aequorin and the green fluorescent protein isolated from *Aequorea forskalea*. *Biochemistry* **17**, 3448–3453.

Rauhut, M. M. (1969). Chemiluminescence from concerted peroxide decomposition reactions. *Acc Chem. Res.* **2**, 80–87.

Rauhut, M. M., Sheehan, D., Clarke, R. A., Roberts, B. G. and Semsel, A. M. (1965a). Chemiluminescence from the reaction of 9-chloro-carbonyl-10-methylacridinium chloride with aqueous hydrogen peroxide. *J. Org. Chem.* **30**, 3587–3592.

Rauhut, M. M., Sheehan, D., Clarke, R. A. and Semsel, A. M. (1965b). Structural criteria for chemiluminescence in acyl peroxide decomposition reaction. *Photochem. Photobiol.* **4**, 1097–1110.

Ribi, M. A., Wei, C. C. and White, E. H. (1972). Energy transfer involving derivatives of luminol. *Tetrahedron* **28**, 481–492.

Roberts, D. R. and White, E. H. (1970). Energy transfer in chemiluminescence. III. Intramolecular triplet–singlet transfer in derivatives of 2,3-dihydrophthalazine-1,4-dione. *J. Am. Chem. Soc.* **92**, 4861–4867.

Roswell, P. F., Paul, V. and White, E. H. (1970). Energy transfer in chemiluminescence II. *J. Am. Chem. Soc.* **92**, 4855–4860.

Rubenstein, K. E., Schneider, R. S. and Ullman, E. F. (1972). 'Homogeneous' enzyme immunoassay. A new immunochemical technique. *Biochem. Biophys. Res. Commun.* **47**, 846–851.

Ruby, E. G. and Nealson, K. H. (1977). A luminous bacterium that emits yellow light. *Science* **196**, 432–434.

Ryzhikov, B. D. (1956). Chemiluminescence of lucigenin. *Bull. Acad. Sci. USSR, Phys. Ser.* **20**, 487–489 (English translation).

Schroeder, H. R., Carrico, R. J. Boguslaski, R. C. and Christner, J. (1976a). Specific reactions with ligand–cofactor conjugates and bacterial luciferase. *Analyt. Biochem.* **72**, 283–292.

Schroeder, H. R., Vogelhut, P. O., Carrico, R. J., Boguslaski, R. C. and Buckler, R. T. (1976b). Competitive protein binding assay for biotin monitored by chemiluminescence. *Analyt. Chem.* **48**, 1933–1937.

Schroeder, H. R., Boguslaski, R. C., Carrico, R. J. and Butler, T. R. (1978). Monitoring specific protein binding reactions with chemiluminescence. *Meth. Enzymol.* **57**, 424–445.

Sharifian, H. A. and Park, S.-M. (1982). Electrogenerated chemiluminescence of several polycyclic aromatic hydrocarbons. *Photochem. Photobiol.* **36**, 83–90.

Shimomura, O. (1979). Structure of the chromophore of *Aequorea* green fluorescent protein. *FEBS Lett.* **104**, 220–222.

Small, E. D., Koka, P. and Lee, J. (1980). Lumazine protein from the bioluminescent bacterium *Photobacterium phosphoreum*. Purification and characterization. *J. Biol. Chem.* **255**, 8804–8810.

Smith, D. S. (1977). Enhancement fluorimmunoassay of thyroxine. *FEBS Lett.* **77**, 25–27.

Sternberg, J. C. (1977). A rate nepholometer for measuring specific protein by immunoprecipitin reaction. *Clin. Chem.* **23**, 1456–1464.

Stryer, L. (1978). Fluorescence energy transfer as a spectroscopic ruler. *A. Rev. Biochem.* **47**, 819–846.

Stryer, L. (1982). Diffusion-enhanced fluorescence energy transfer. *A. Rev. Biophys. Bioeng.* **11**, 203–222.

Stryer, L. and Haugland, R. P. (1967). Energy transfer: a spectroscopic ruler. *Proc. Natn. Acad. Sci. U.S.A.* **58**, 719–726.

Tiemann, D. L. (1970). Nature's toy train, the railroad worm. *Nat. Hist. Mag.* **138**, 56–67.

Tomita, G. and Rabinowitch, E. (1962). Excitation energy transfer between pigments in photosynthetic cells. *Biophys. J.* **2**, 483–499.

Tscharner, V. von and Bailey, I. A. (1983). Non-invasive, kinetic measurements of [^{3}H]nitrendipine binding to isolated rat mycocytes by condensed phase radioluminescence. *FEBS Lett.* **162**, 185–188.

Ullman, E. F. and Khanna, P. L. (1981). Fluorescence excitation transfer immunoassay (FETI). *Meth. Enzymol.* **74C**, 28–60.

Ullman, E. F., Schwarzberg, M. and Rubenstein, K. E. (1976). Fluorescent excitation transfer immunoassay. A general method for determination of antigens. *J. Biol. Chem.* **251**, 4172–4178.

Velick, S. F. (1958). Fluorescence spectra and polarization of glyceraldehyde-3-phosphate and lactic dehydrogenase coenzyme complexes. *J. Biol. Chem.* **233**, 1455–1467.

Velick, S. F., Parker, C. W. and Eisen, H. N. (1960). Excitation energy transfer and the quantitative study of the antibody hapten reaction. *Proc. Natn. Acad. Sci. U.S.A.* **46**, 1470–1482.

Vernon, T., Alexander, O. L., Glazer, N. and Stryer, L. (1982). Fluorescent phycobiliprotein conjugates for analyses of cells and molecules. *J. Cell Biol.* **93**, 981–986.

Vervoori, J., O'Kane, D. J., Carreira, L. A. and Lee, J. (1983). Identification of a lumazine protein from *Photobacterium leiognathi* by coherent anti-Stokes Raman spectroscopy. *Photochem. Photobiol.* **37**, 117–119.

Visser, A. J. W. G. and Lee. J. (1980). Lumazine protein from the bioluminescent bacterium *Photobacterium phosphoreum*. A fluorescence study of the protein–ligand equilibrium. *Biochemistry* **19**, 4366–4372.

Visser, A. J. W. G. and Lee, J. (1982). Association between lumazine protein and bacterial luciferase: direct demonstration from the decay of the lumazine emission anisotropy. *Biochemistry* **21**, 2218–2226.

Ward, W. W. (1979). Energy transfer processes in bioluminescence. *Photochem. Photobiol. Rev.* **4**, 1–58.

Ward, W. W. and Cormier, M. J. (1976). *In vitro* energy transfer in *Renilla* bioluminescence. *J. Phys. Chem.* **80**, 2289–2291.

Ward, W. W. and Cormier, M. J. (1978). Energy transfer via protein–protein interaction in *Renilla* bioluminescence. *Photochem. Photobiol.* **27**, 389–396.

Ward, W. W. and Cormier, M. J. (1979). An energy transfer protein in coelenterate bioluminescence. Characterization of the *Renilla* green–fluorescent protein. *J. Biol. Chem.* **254**, 781–788.

Ward, W. W., Prentice, H. J., Roth, A. F., Cody, C. W. and Reeves, S. C. (1982). Spectral perturbation of the *Aequorea* green fluorescent protein. *Photochem. Photobiol.* **35**, 803–808.

Weeks, I., Beheshti, I., McCapra, F., Campbell, A. K. and Woodhead, J. S. (1983a). Acridinium esters as high specific activity labels in immunoassay. *Clin. Chem.* **29**, 1474–1479.

Weeks, I., Campbell, A. K. and Woodhead, J. S. (1983b). Two-site immunochemiluminometric assay for human α_1-fetoprotein. *Clin. Chem.* **29**, 1480–1483.

White, E. H. and Roswell, D. F. (1967). Intramolecular energy transfer in chemiluminescence. *J. Am. Chem. Soc.* **89**, 3944–3945.

White, E. H. and Roswell, D. F. (1970). The chemiluminescence of organic hydrazides. *Acc. Chem. Res.* **3**, 54–62.

White, E. H., Roberts, D. R. and Roswell, D. F. (1969). Energy transfer in chemiluminescence. In *Molecular Luminescence* (E. C. Lin, ed.), Benjamin, New York, pp. 479–492.

White, E. H., Maino, J. D., Watkins, C. J. and Breaux, E. J. (1974). Chemically produced excited states. *Angew. Chem. Int. Edn* **13**, 229–243.

Alternative Immunoassays
Edited by W. P. Collins
© 1985 John Wiley & Sons Ltd

CHAPTER 11

Fluoroimmunoassays and phosphoroimmunoassays

A.M. SIDKI and J. LANDON

Department of Chemical Pathology,
St Bartholomew's Hospital,
London EC1A 7BE, UK

---

1. INTRODUCTION

As the name implies, immunoassays are analytical procedures based on an immunological reaction. They depend upon the reversible, non-covalent binding of the analyte to be measured (the antigen, Ag) by specific antibodies (Ab) in a reaction which obeys the law of mass action:

$$Ag + Ab \underset{k_2}{\overset{k_1}{\rightleftharpoons}} Ag : Ab$$

$$\text{(free fraction)} \qquad \text{(bound fraction)}$$

At equilibrium some of the free reactants will be combining with a rate constant, k_1, to form more of the antigen : antibody complex while some of the complex will be dissociating, with a rate constant, k_2, to give free analyte and antibodies. Such assays owe their widespread and rapidly increasing use to the specificity inherent with immunological reactions, their potential sensitivity, their practicality and, in particular, their wide applicability.

Immunoassays can be categorized into those in which no labelled reactant is required, those employing labelled antigen as a tracer and others in which specific antibodies are labelled. Despite their relative simplicity, easy adaptation to existing laboratory instruments and extensive use for the assay of several serum proteins and glycoproteins, non-labelled immunoassays have severe limitations. Thus, because of the need to form extensive antigen : antibody complexes for these to be detectable, they are applicable only to large molecules present in relatively high concentrations. Furthermore, specificity depends solely on the antiserum used and the assays are prone to give spurious results in antigen excess due to the prozone phenomenon.

The introduction of radioimmunoassays (RIA), which are based on the use of isotopically labelled antigen, has proved an important milestone. They enable the assay of haptens, such as drugs and the thyroid and steroid hormones, as well as large molecules. Both sensitivity and specificity are markedly improved and there are no longer problems with antigen excess. The labelled analyte acts as a tracer to enable determination of the distribution of total analyte (labelled and unlabelled) between the antibody-bound and free fractions. Provided that the amounts of tracer and of antiserum are kept constant and in limited concentration, the percentage of the counts present in the bound fraction is inversely related to the initial concentration of unlabelled analyte in the samples and standards being assayed. More recently a new type of immunoassay, termed immunoradiometric assay (IRMA), has been developed based on the use of isotopically labelled specific antibodies. It offers certain advantages over RIA but, for reasons of space, IRMA and its non-isotopic equivalents will not be considered further in this paper (see Chapters 3, 5, 9 and 13 in this volume).

The dominant reactant in all types of immunoassay is the antibody because it is this which, in large part, determines both the specificity and sensitivity that can be achieved. The isotope in a RIA is employed only as a tracer and many other labels are proving suitable in addition to gamma - and beta-emitting radionuclides. To date these have included the following: free radicals; enzymes, coenzymes and enzyme inhibitors; viruses; proteins and glycoproteins; gold and silver sols; red blood cells, latex and other particles; and fluorescent, phosphorescent, chemiluminescent and bioluminescent molecules.

Considerable confusion is inevitable unless a common terminology is introduced that, for example, clearly distinguishes whether what is being referred to is a RIA to measure the concentration of an enzyme or an immunoassay employing an enzyme as the label. The terminology and acronyms used should give regard to that suggested by the originators and the term radioimmunoassay (RIA) has been extended to enzymoimmunoassays (EIA), fluoroimmunoassays (FIA) and phosphoroimmunoassays (PhIA), which are immunoassays employing antigen labelled with an enzyme, a fluorophore or a phosphore respectively. It would also seem correct to extend the use of the term immunoradiometric assays (IRMA) to immunofluorometric (IFMA) and immunophosphorometric (IPhMA) assays if specific labelled antibodies are used. Finally, it seems reasonable to refer to separation and non-separation assays (in preference to the commonly used but less explicit terms, homogeneous and heterogeneous) for those non-isotopic immunoassays which include and those which do not require a separation step respectively.

This chapter will summarize the basis of fluorescence and phosphorescence. Then, using the anticonvulsant drug, primidone, as an example, it will describe some of the separation and non-separation FIA and PhIA developed in our laboratories. Finally, their advantages and disadvantages will be compared briefly with those of RIA and some other non-isotopic immunoassays (NIIA).

2. BASIS OF FLUORESCENCE AND PHOSPHORESCENCE

Absorption of a photon of appropriate energy (wavelength) can excite a molecule from its usual ground state (S_0) to a higher electronic singlet state (S_1, S_2, S_3, etc.) in which the electrons remain paired but an outer electron is promoted to a higher energy level (Fig. 1). This state is extremely unstable and the molecule rapidly loses much of the excess vibrational and electronic energy by non-radiative means, such as release of heat, and relaxes to the lowest vibrational level of the first excited singlet state (S_1).

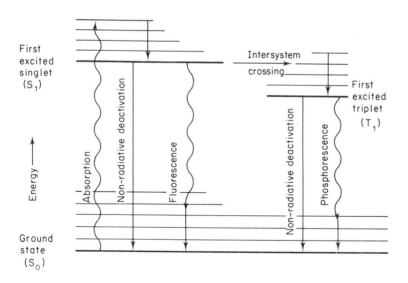

Fig. 1. A Jablonski diagram illustrating the events involved in fluorescence and phosphorescence

The luminescent properties of the molecule depend upon what happens next. Most molecules will return to the ground state without emitting light, the excess energy being lost by 'internal conversion', by various quenching processes or via 'intersystem crossing' to the first excited triplet electronic state (T_1 in Fig. 1). Alternatively, one of two light-emitting processes can occur, namely fluorescence, in which a photon of light is emitted as the molecule moves from the singlet (S_1) to the ground state (S_0), or phosphorescence, in which emission of a photon of light occurs as the molecule relaxes from the triplet (T_1) to the ground state.

Fluorescence may be extremely efficient with a high quantum yield (which expresses the ratio of the number of emitted photons to the number of exciting photons. It is also usually relatively rapid, characterized by a first order decay with a lifetime measured in nanoseconds. Also, while the emitted photon must always be of longer wavelength (i.e. have less energy) than the exciting photon, the difference between the two, the Stokes' shift, is often small. As an example, the quantum yield of fluorescein approaches the maximum possible value of unity, the time between excitation and emission is about 5 ns and the Stokes' shift is less than 30 nm (excitation maxima about 492 nm; emission maxima about 517 nm).

By contrast, phosphorescence is very inefficient with a low quantum yield and, because of the transfer from S_1 to T_1, is characterized by very long radiative lifetimes (ranging from milliseconds to seconds) and a large Stokes' shift. As an example, the quantum yield of the phosphore, erythrosin, is less than 0.01, its radiative lifetime is several hundred milliseconds and its Stokes' shift about 150 nm (excitation maxima about 540 nm; emission maxima about 690 nm). Because of the long radiative lifetime, the molecule has a very high probability of losing excess energy by non-radiative transitions such as internal conversion or photodecomposition or quenching of the triplet state (the means by which oxygen is particularly effective in preventing phosphorescence).

3.   EXAMPLES OF FLUOROIMMUNOASSAYS AND PHOSPHOROIMMUNOASSAYS

3.1. Fluoroimmunoassays

Our department has been actively engaged in developing novel forms of FIA and applying them to more than 40 analytes for nearly a decade. The subject has recently been reviewed (Smith et al., 1981) and only two examples will be given.

3.1.1. Separation fluoroimmunoassay for primidone

The separation step can serve two functions in a FIA: first, to separate the antibody bound and free fractions and, second, to enable removal of any endogenous fluorophores or other factors present in the sample which might interfere with end-point measurement. This second function enables the assay of large serum samples and markedly increases sensitivity.

The development of a magnetizable particle, separation FIA for primidone (Sidki *et al.*, 1983) will serve as an example. Antisera were raised in sheep by immunization with a suitable immunogen and coupled, by the cyanogen bromide technique, to magnetizable particles. An amino derivative of primidone was reacted directly with fluorescein isothiocyanate (FITC) to give the label (P-FITC). The assay involved the serial addition of 5 μl of sample, or standard, 100 μl of P-FITC (580 nmol l^{-1}) and 100 μl of solid-phase antiserum (10 g l^{-1}) into disposable polystyrene tubes. After a few minutes incubation at ambient temperature with constant mixing, 1 ml of diluent buffer was added, the particles sedimented on a magnet and the supernates (containing the free fraction and all interfering factors) decanted to waste. The bound fraction was released by addition of an elution reagent, the particles again sedimented magnetically and the fluorescence of the eluates determined directly in a fluorimeter. Finally, a dose–response curve was constructed by plotting the percentage of total fluorescence that was antibody bound against the concentration of serum-based standards (Fig. 2).

3.1.2. Non-separation fluoroimmunoassay for primidone

The use of FITC as a label has enabled the development of several different non-separation FIAs for both haptens and large molecules. Of these, assays based on the application of fluorescence polarization for haptens have proved the most successful and formed the basis of the Abbott TDX system. This department was the first to use fluorescence polarization in a clinical context (Watson *et al.*, 1976; McGregor *et al.*, 1978) and uses this technique for the initial assessment of virtually all the antisera we raise against haptens. This reflects the simplicity of fluorescence polarization which depends upon the large increases in signal that occur when a fluorescein-labelled hapten is bound by specific antibodies against the hapten.

In the development of a polarization fluoroimmunoassay (PFIA) for primidone, the same antiserum and tracer were used as above. A 50-fold dilution of serum sample or standard is prepared in a pre-treatment reagent comprising pepsin in 100 mmol l^{-1} HCl (10 mg l^{-1}). Fifty microlitres of this solution is pipetted into a disposable glass cuvette containing 1.5 ml of sheep anti-primidone serum (diluted 1 in 4000) pre-mixed with fluorescein-labelled primidone in borate buffer containing gelatin and sodium azide. After a few

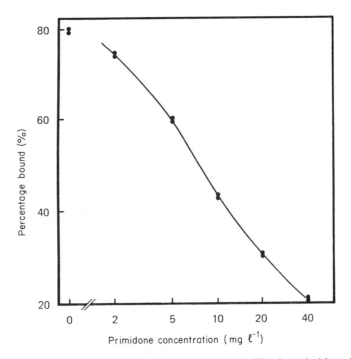

Fig. 2. The dose–response curve obtained in a separation FIA for primidone based on
the use of antibodies covalently linked to magnetizable particles

minutes incubation, equilibrium is reached and fluorescence polarization is
measured directly and a dose–response curve constructed (Fig. 3). This
covers the same clinically relevant range as the separation FIA and it can be
seen that antibody binding of the tracer (in the zero standard) results in a
marked rise in signal that falls as progressively more unlabelled primidone is
present—and competes for the antibody binding sites.

The PFIA are extremely quick and simple to perform. However, like all
non-separation FIA, they are prone to a number of interferences—including
endogenous fluorescence, light scattering, inner-filter effects and non-specific
binding of the tracer by albumin or other serum proteins. This is illustrated by
a series of experiments summarized in Table 1. Normal human serum and
even buffer alone gave a significant fluorescence signal while a patient's
sample with hyperbilirubinaemia gave a large signal (about one-third that of
the fluorescein label). The situation was made more difficult by the fact that
normal serum and, in particular, serum from the icteric patient significantly
decreased the fluorescence signal of the fluorescein. Such problems are
overcome by the separation step in the separation FIA and the Abbott TDX

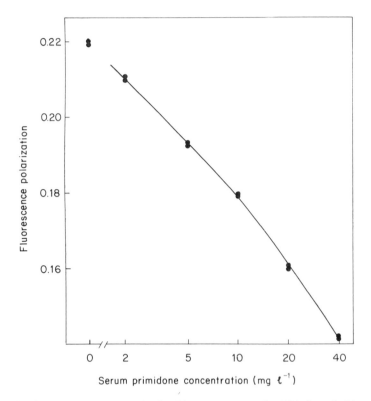

Fig. 3. The dose–response curve obtained in a non-separation FIA for primidone based on the change in fluorescence polarization when P-FITC is bound by antibodies

system attempts to overcome them by routine inclusion of a sample blank and application of a correction factor. However, we have found that even the latter does not avoid erroneous results being obtained if very haemolyzed or jaundiced samples are assayed by polarization FIA.

3.2. Phosphoroimmunoassays

In Chapters 7, 12 and 13 of this book, time-resolved fluorometry has been advocated as an elegant means of avoiding sample interference in FIA, thereby obtaining a marked improvement in sensitivity. In that approach a rare earth chelate is employed as the label and time-resolution used to 'blank out' sample effects. However, the chemistry of the rare earth chelates is complex and the LKB methods involve a separation step—which adds to the complexity and time taken to perform an assay.

Table 1. Studies with fluorescein and erythrosin

	Fluorescence signal (arbitrary units)	Phosphoresc-ence signal (arbitrary units)
(a) *Exitation at 492 nm and emission determined at 517 nm*		
Buffer alone	1.5	
Buffer + 100 μl normal human serum (NHS)	5	
Buffer + 100 μl icteric serum†	35	
Buffer + fluorescein (10 nmol l^{-1})	115	
Buffer + 100 μl NHS + fluorescein	85	
Buffer + 100 μl icteric serum + fluorescein	73	
(b) *Excitation at 540 nm and emission determined at 690 nm*		
Buffer alone		0
Buffer + 100 μl normal human serum (NHS)		0
Buffer + 100 μl icteric serum †		0
Buffer + erythrosin (100 nmol l^{-1})		255
Buffer + 100 μl NHS + erythrosin		255
Buffer + 100 μl icteric serum + erythrosin		255

† Icteric serum had a bilirubin level of 530 μmol l^{-1}

We have adopted a different approach to avoid sample interference while retaining the simplicity of labelling and end-point detection that characterizes FIA. Phosphoroimmunoassays (PhIA) are a new generation of immunoassay techniques developed in our department. The present assays employ the phosphorescence probe, erythrosin, as the label and depend upon measuring its long lifetime emission in a time-resolved luminescence spectrometer. The large Stokes' shift (150 nm), the longer wavelengths involved as compared with fluorescein and, in particular, time-resolved detection (Fig. 4) enable complete rejection of short-lived background signals, including those from endogenous fluorophores or light-scattering components of biological fluids. Furthermore, the use of erythrosin isothiocyanate (EITC) enables application of the same chemistries developed to label molecules with FITC.

Table 1 illustrates the effective way in which this approach overcomes background interference. Thus, in an identical set of experiments to those used to study fluorescein, it was found that neither normal nor icteric sera give a signal and nor do they alter the signal given by erythrosin. However, it should be noted that the amount of erythrosin used was 10 times that of fluorescein.

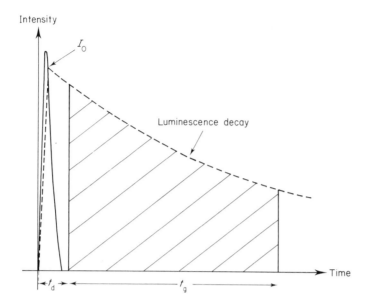

Fig. 4. Representation of the events involved in time-resolved phosphorescence measurement. t_d is the delay from the beginning of the pulse to the beginning of observation; t_g is the gate width of the detector (the signal collected during t_g is integrated). The broken line indicates a build-up of luminescence signal to a maximum, I_0, and then exponential decay

3.2.1. Phosphorescent-labelling and phosphorometry in solution

In the development of the present range of PhIA, erythrosin (tetraiodofluorescein) was chosen as the phosphorescent label. Among several advantages, it exhibits phosphorescence and delayed fluorescence with an appropriate lifetime in the microsecond range; it can be prepared easily from fluorescein and is available commercially as the reactive isothiocyanate derivative—which enables direct coupling to primary or secondary amine groups exactly as with FITC; and, because of its luminescence spectra, which lie in the visible region (Fig. 5) and large Stokes' shift, absorption of light by serum components is avoided and inner filter error markedly reduced.

Two factors may have delayed the application of phosphores to immunoassay: the commonly held view that cryogenic or solid-state conditions are necessary for analytical phosphorometry and the knowledge that oxygen effectively quenches the triplet state. However, it is now known that useful phosphorescent signals can be obtained in fluid media at room temperature (Miller, 1981) provided that oxygen quenching is avoided. To date oxygen is usually removed by freeze–pump–thaw cycling or by bubbling of solutions

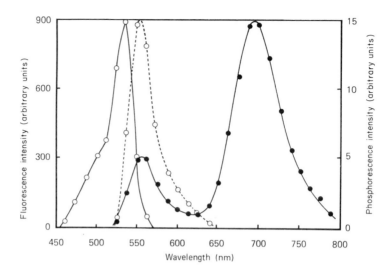

Fig. 5. The fluorescence and phosphorescence excitation and emission maxima for erythrosin. O–O represents the fluorescence and phosphorescence excitation spectra; O---O represents the prompt fluorescence; ●–● represents the delayed fluorescence (lower intensity peak with similar spectra to that of prompt fluorescence) and the phosphorescence which appears at longer wavelengths (peak at 690 nm). The time-resolved measurements were made with delay and gate time settings of 40 and 300 μs respectively

with nitrogen or argon for several minutes. Such tedious procedures would clearly be inappropriate to many hundred clinical samples.

Simple means of *in situ* chemical deoxygenization were studied. Various chemical methods for removing oxygen are known (Willis, 1964; Ebsworth *et al.*, 1973), but most are too harsh for inclusion with immunological reactions or involve coloured reagents that could interfere with luminescence measurements. Fortunately, various salts of the sulphur oxyacids, in particular sodium sulphite, were found useful in enabling a good phosphorescence signal to be produced at room temperature in the open atmosphere—by rapidly reducing the oxygen concentration of the aqueous solution to virtually zero (*Gmelins Handbuch*, 1963; Ebsworth *et al.*, 1973).

A Perkin-Elmer Model LS-5 luminescence spectrophotometer was used for time-resolved measurements. The delay time (t_d), which is the time between the pulse of exciting light and the start of measurement, was selected at 40 μs and the gate time (t_g), which is the time interval over which the signal is subsequently measured, was set at 300 μs. The excitation and emission wavelengths were set to correspond to the excitation and emission spectral peaks for erythrosin phosphorescence of 536 and 690 nm respectively with a monochromator bandpass of 5 and 20 nm respectively. Assays were performed in polystyrene disposable tubes (Sarstedt 484, 55 mm × 12 mm), which were placed directly in the cuvette compartment of the instrument by means of a special adaptor (Kamel *et al.*, 1980).

3.2.2. *Separation phosphoroimmunoassay for primidone*

One of the advantages of PhIA is the ease with which it can be developed based on a pre-existing separation FIA. Thus, in the development of a magnetizable particle, separation PhIA for primidone, the same particles and antisera were used as described earlier. Erythrosin-labelled primidone (P-EITC) was prepared by the direct reaction of 4-aminophenyl primidone with erythrosin isothiocyanate and purified by thin-layer chromatography. The assay was also very similar in its initial stages involving the sequential addition of serum samples (or standard), 100 μl of P-EITC (930 nmol l^{-1}) and 100 μl of solid-phase antiserum suspension (25 g l^{-1}) followed by incubation at room temperature with constant mixing until equilibrium had been attained (Fig. 6).

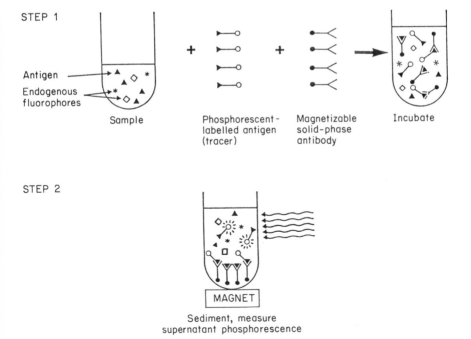

Fig. 6. Representation of a separation phosphoroimmunoassay procedure

Thereafter, all that was required was to add 1.3 ml of diluent buffer containing sodium sulphate (12 g l^{-1}), sediment the magnetizable particles and bound fraction by means of a magnet and measure the phosphorescence signal of the supernates, containing the free fractions, directly. Finally, a dose–response curve is constructed by plotting the percentage of the total phosphorescence present in the free fraction against the concentration of primidone in the human serum-based standards (Fig. 7). It can be seen that, as with all previous dose-response curves for this anticonvulsant, the clinically relevant range of values is covered.

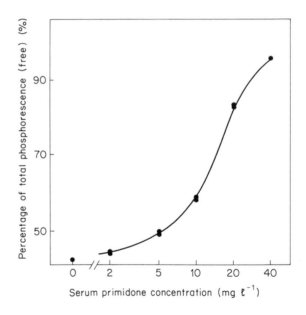

Fig. 7. The dose–response curve obtained in a separation PhIA for primidone based on the use of antibodies covalently linked to magnetizable particles

This assay is simpler than its FIA counterpart because the lack of sample interference enables the phosphorescence of the free fraction to be measured directly—rather than having to discard the free fraction with the serum interfering factors and then elute the bound fraction from the magnetizable particles prior to end-point measurement. Indeed, so simple and rapid is the step necessary to sediment the particles from the light path that this type of assay compares favourably with non-separation PhIA.

3.2.3. Non-separation phosphoroimmunoassay for primidone

It proved easy to develop a non-separation PhIA for primidone based on the finding that the binding of P-EITC by any of a number of antisera to the drug caused a marked decrease in phosphorescence. The quenching PhIA is based on the unlabelled hapten, in a patient's sample or standard, competing for the limited number of antibody binding sites. As a result, less of the labelled primidone is bound and the phosphorescence signal is enhanced. The assay is further simplified by pre-mixing the labelled primidone with the appropriate dilution of antiserum—made possible by the rapid k_2 which characterizes hapten : antibody binding.

To 1.5 ml of a pool of P-EITC (60 nmol l^{-1}) and a 1 in 270 dilution of sheep anti-primidone serum in diluent buffer containing sodium sulphite (12 g l^{-1}) is added 5 µl of sample or standard. After a few minutes at room temperature, phosphorescence is read and a dose–response curve constructed (Fig. 8) which covers the clinically relevant range.

This simple non-separation quenching type of PhIA has proved applicable to a wide range of haptens. Thus, antibodies against barbiturates, carbamazepine, gentamicin, theophylline, thyroxine and cortisol were all found to quench the phosphorescence of the erythrosin-labelled analyte and such quenching was rapidly reversed by the addition of the unlabelled hapten.

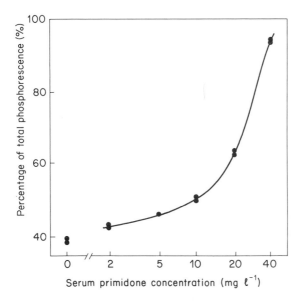

Fig. 8. The dose-response curve obtained in a non-separation PhIA for primidone based on the quenching of the phosphorescence signal when P-EITC is bound by antibodies

4. COMPARISON WITH OTHER IMMUNOASSAYS

RIA provides the reference technique with which all types of NIIA must be compared. In addition, FIA and PhIA must be compared with the many other non-isotopic procedures and the various factors influencing choice of label are listed in Table 2.

Table 2. Factors influencing the choice of label for immunoassays

1.	Potential emotive bias against use
2.	Simplicity of labelling and the immunogenicity of the labelled reactant
3.	Shelf-life of the labelled reactant
4.	Ability to develop non-separation immunoassays
5.	Speed, simplicity, precision and sensitivity of end-point detection†
6.	Liability to interference by factors present in biological fluids†

†Factors 5 and 6 help determine the sensitivity that can be obtained

4.1 Freedom from any health hazard or emotive bias

The use of ^{125}I-labelled antigen in a RIA does not carry any health hazard provided that elementary safety precautions are followed. However, there is a potential risk to health during radioiodinations, legislation relating to the disposal of radioactive waste is tedious to comply with in some countries and there is an increasing emotive bias against the use of radionuclides. FIA and PhIA, like virtually all forms of NIIA other than those employing a virus as the label, avoid these problems.

4.2. Simplicity of labelling

The preparation of the labelled antigen for use in FIA and PhIA is probably simpler than for any other kind of immunoassay. Furthermore, the gentle conditions required for labelling help ensure that the immunogenicity of the labelled analyte is unimpaired and, therefore, that assays can be developed in which antisera do not distinguish between the labelled and unlabelled compound. In comparison, radioiodination is much more complex and potentially damaging and one of the reasons why we have delayed using rare earth chelates is the complexity of the chemistries involved.

4.3. Shelf-life of the labelled antigen

Analytes labelled with a fluorophore or phosphore have a virtually indefinite shelf-life provided that they are stored correctly. For example, we have a sample of fluorescein-labelled thyroxine prepared eight years ago that still retains full immunogenicity. Nearly all types of non-isotopically labelled molecules share this advantage with its potential for markedly reducing manufacturing, quality assurance and distribution costs as compared with RIA kits—which have a useful life usually measured in weeks.

4.4. Ability to develop non-separation immunoassays

None of the non-labelled immunoassays require a separation step whereas most assays employing an isotope as a label must include such a step. FIA and PhIA, like most other NIIA, can be developed in which antibody binding changes the nature of the signal, decreases the signal (as in the direct quenching PhIA described earlier) or increases the signal (as in fluorescence polarization). Examples are given in Table 3 and there is no doubt that the variety of non-separation approaches possible with FIA and PhIA is greater than with other forms of NIIA, including EIA.

Table 3. Types of non-separation immunoassay

A.	Non-labelled immunoassays
B.	Immunoassays employing labelled antigens
	Antibody binding alters the signal
	Antibody binding decreases the signal Direct quenching immunoassays Energy transfer immunoassays
	Antibody binding increases the signal Direct enhancement immunoassays Indirect quenching immunoassays Polarization fluoroimmunoassays
C.	Immunoassays employing labelled antibodies

Avoidance of a separation step is a considerable advantage since it simplifies and significantly shortens an assay and may improve precision. One interesting observation is that while only a few antisera against gentamicin significantly quenched the fluorescent signal of FITC-labelled gentamicin, all decreased the phosphorescent signal given by EITC–gentamicin.

4.5. Simplicity, speed, sensitivity and precision of end-point measurement

Phosphorescence and fluorescence can be measured directly within a few seconds with a precision considerably greater than that for a gamma-emitting isotope or an enzyme. However, the low quantum efficiency of erythrosin as compared with fluorescein significantly reduced the sensitivity that could be attained with conventional instrumentation. Use of a photon counter would considerably enhance sensitivity and it remains to be seen whether more efficient phosphores than erythrosin can be found.

4.6. Liability to sample interference

The single most important advantage of an isotopic label, such as ^{125}I, is the freedom from interference. Thus, nothing present in biological fluids either increases or decreases the number of counts recorded and it is this which, in large part, ensures the sensitivity of RIA. Most other forms of immunoassay are subject to sample interference—rheumatoid factor or complement factor Clq may cause erroneous results with non-labelled immunoassays; EIA may be influenced by the presence of endogenous enzymes or enzyme inhibitors; and FIA, as discussed earlier, is prone to a variety of non-specific effects.

Time-resolved fluorescence avoids such problems and an encouraging feature of PhIA is the absence of sample interference when used in the time-resolved mode. As a result, large sample volumes can be employed and, thereby, sensitivity improved. Nonetheless, the sensitivity currently achieved does not match that of RIA or of time-resolved FIA using a rare earth chelate as the label.

5. CONCLUSIONS

At this moment in time the various types of immunoassay have a complementary role and there is no single ideal label for use in all immunoassays. Thus, the choice should be based on the analyte to be measured, the purpose for which the measurement will be made and where the assay is to be performed. For example, an assay designed to detect the β subunit of human choriogonadotrophin in the diagnosis of pregnancy should probably differ from an assay developed to quantitate this glycoprotein accurately in the monitoring of treatment for a choriocarcinoma. Likewise, immunoassays designed for the developing world may well differ from those in a country with full access to modern, expensive equipment.

In general, non-labelled immunoassay would seem to be the technique of choice for the specific serum proteins and glycoproteins with RIA (and, in the near future, time-resolved FIA) being preferred for situations where sensitivity and accurate quantitation are required (such as for many hormones and for neonatal screening when sample volumes must be limited). EIA would seem ideal for the many situations requiring a plus or minus answer, because of the potential for visual or simple colorimetric end-point measurements. However, recent experience with polarization FIA indicates that this approach is preferable to non-separation EIA for therapeutic drug monitoring. It would seem that, in the near future, FIA and PhIA may replace RIA for such analytes as thyroxine and cortisol.

REFERENCES

Ebsworth, E. A. V., Connor, J. A., and Turner, J. J. (1973). Oxygen. In *Comprehensive Inorganic Chemistry*, Vol. 2 (J. C. Bailar, H. J. Emeleus, R. Nyholm and A. F. Trotman-Dickenson, eds), Pergamon, Oxford, pp. 685–794.

Gmelin's Handbuch (1963). *Gmelin's Handbuch*, System Number 9, *Schwefel*, Teil B, Lieferung 3, Verlag Chemie, Weinheim, pp. 1293–1514.

Kamel, R. S., Landon, J., and Smith, D. S. (1980). Magnetizable solid-phase fluoroimmunoassay of phenytoin in disposable test tubes. *Clin. Chem.* **26**, 1281–1284.

McGregor, A. R., Crookall-Greening, J. O., Landon, J., and Smith, D. S. (1978). Polarization fluoroimmunoassay of phenytoin. *Clin. Chim. Acta* **83**, 161–166.

Miller, J. N. (1981). Room temperature phosphorimetry—a promising trace analysis method. *Trends Analyt. Chem.* **1**, 31–34.

Sidki, A. M., Rowell, F. J. and Landon, J. (1983). Direct determination of primidone in serum or plasma by a magnetizable solid-phase fluoroimmunoassay. *Ann. Clin. Biochem.* **20**, 227–232.

Smith, D. S., Al-Hakiem, M. H. H. and Landon, J. (1981). A review of fluoroimmunoassay and immunofluorometric assay. *Ann. Clin. Biochem.* **18**, 253–274.

Watson, R. A. A., Landon, J., Shaw, E. J. and Smith, D. S. (1976). Polarization fluoroimmunoasay of gentamicin. *Clin. Chim. Acta* **73**, 51–55.

Willis, A. T. (1964). *Anaerobic Bacteriology in Clinical Medicine*, Butterworth, London.

Alternative Immunoassays
Edited by W. P. Collins
© 1985 John Wiley & Sons Ltd

CHAPTER 12

Time-resolved fluorometry in immunoassay

T. Lovgren,† I. Hemmilä,† K. Pettersson† and P. Halonen‡

† Wallac Biochemical Laboratory,
PO Box 10,
SF-20101 Turku 10,
Finland

‡Department of Virology,
University of Turku,
SF-20520 Turku 52,
Finland

1. INTRODUCTION

At present radioimmunoassay is still one of the most widely used analytical procedures. It is, however, continuously challenged by a number of non-isotopic techniques, e.g. several enzyme-, chemiluminescence- or fluorescence-based immunoassays. Because of the potential sensitivity obtained in the quantitation of fluorescent molecules they could be an ideal choice for future labels. Until recently their usefulness has, however, been limited by the high background fluorescence always present in the measurements, which seriously limits the sensitivity of the assay. The problem has been overcome by the use of time-resolved fluorescence and labels with a long fluorescent decay time. This chapter reviews the measurement of lanthanides with high sensitivity using time-resolved fluorescence, and their use as labels, in immunoassays where high sensitivity is required.

2. TIME-RESOLVED MEASUREMENTS AND FLUORESCENT LABELS

Time-resolved fluorometry is a fluorescence technique in which the lifetime of the emission which occurs after pulsed light excitation is followed at a certain wavelength. The characteristics of the observed fluorescence depend on the properties of the fluorophore excited by the pulsed light source. In this respect at least two of the parameters are important, namely the amount of excitation energy released, which affects the wavelength of the emitted light, and the speed of the energy transition in the fluorophore, which affects the decay time of the emitted light (Vallarino et al., 1979).

Immunoassay methods employing conventional fluorescent labels have been used quite extensively, although they never achieved the high sensitivity of radiolabelled assays (Landon and Kamel, 1981). However, a number of simple fluorescence-based non-separation principles have been developed for measuring analytes present in concentrations which do not require high sensitivity. The main reason for limited sensitivity of the fluorescent labels is the high background fluorescence associated with such materials as plastic and glass in the instrument and proteins in the sample. In order to overcome the limitation set by background fluorescence the time-resolved assay principle is applied (Soini and Hemmilä, 1979; Hemmilä et al., 1984). The half-life of the background fluorescence is in the order of 10 ns. Consequently, if the actual measuring time of a specific fluorescent signal in the time-resolved mode starts after the background fluorescence has decayed, an increase in sensitivity is postulated. The basic principle of the measurement is shown in Fig. 1 (see also Chapters 7 and 13, in this volume).

In order to be able to utilize the benefits of time-resolved fluorescence when applied to immunoassays, the labels should be fluorophores with a fluorescence lifetime considerably longer than that of the components giving rise to the background signal. In Table 1 the fluorescence half-life of some proteins, commonly used fluorescence labels and europium chelates are listed. It is evident that the decay time of commonly used fluorescent labels, such as dansyl chloride and fluorescein isothiocyanate, is of the same order of magnitude as that of, for example, proteins. Consequently, the use of a time-resolved technique will not bring any improvement when these labels are used. On the other hand the fluorescent half-life of certain lanthanide chelates, such as europium chelates, is some five to six orders of magnitude longer than that of conventional fluorescent labels (Vallarino et al., 1979). The emission from europium chelates can thus be distinguished from the background fluorescence with a short decay time by using a time-resolved fluorometer with properly selected delay, counting and cycle times (Soini and Kojola, 1983).

The decay time and intensity of europium fluorescence is very much dependent on the structure of the ligands which chelate europium and on the physical environment around the europium ion which emits the light (Hemmilä et al., 1984). Obviously these parameters have to be carefully controlled before europium is used as a label in immunoassays. In addition, methods have to be devised to bind the label to one of the immunoreactive components of the assay.

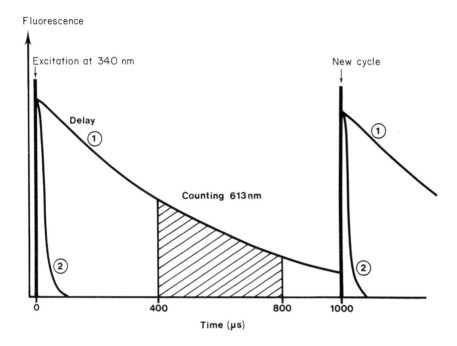

Fig. 1. Measurement principle of time-resolved fluorescence. The cycle time is 1 ms and pulsed excitation less than 1 µs occurs at the beginning of each cycle. The delay time after the pulsed excitation is 400 µs and the actual counting time within the cycle has the same duration. The total measurement time is 1 s. Curve 1 represents the fluorescence of the europium chelate and curve 2 the background fluorescence (actual decay time less than 1 µs)

Table 1. Fluorescence decay time of some fluorophores and proteins

Substance	Decay time (ns)
Human serum albumin	4.1
Cytochrome c	3.5
Globin (haemoglobin)	3.0
Fluorescein isothiocynate	4.5
Dansyl chloride	14
Europium chelates	10^3–10^6

3. MEASUREMENT OF EUROPIUM WITH HIGH SENSITIVITY

Although the fluorescence emission originates from the europium ion, the surrounding organic ligands have a very important function in the process (Crosby et al., 1961). The model for the fluorescence of a europium chelate has been described as a sequence of four steps (Vallarino et al., 1979): (i) excitation of the organic ligand; (ii) intersystem crossing within the excited ligand (energy is transferred from the singlet excited state to a triplet excited state of the ligand); (iii) intramolecular energy transfer (energy is transferred from the triplet excited state of a ligand to the resonance levels of the europium ion); (iv) light emission from the europium ion.

The emission spectrum of the europium ion fluorescence will thus be a characteristic of the metal ion itself, while the half-life and intensity of the fluorescence depend on the environment in which the ion is present, including the properties of the ligand. Any change in the environment can thus be expected to influence both the half-life and intensity.

Different β-diketones ($R^1COCH_2COR^2$) chelate europium ions and possess the properties required for excitation (Hemmilä et al., 1984). Different fluorescence intensities are observed by varying the nature of the functional groups in positions R^1 and R^2. Furthermore, the intensity is affected by the nature of the solvent around the chelated europium ion. In water solutions a quenching effect is observed due to loss of energy as heat from the excited complex to the surrounding water molecules. As the europium quantitation in immunoassays occurs in a water solution, a measuring solution had to be designed to dissolve the β-diketone required for energy absorption and transfer, and simultaneously to protect the ion from quenching by water molecules. This objective was achieved with a non-ionic detergent, Triton X-100, which dissolves the sparingly soluble organic component in the micellar phase and excludes the quenching water from the chelated europium ion. The insulation from the solvent has been further optimized by the addition of a synergistic agent, trioctylphosphine oxide, to the europium chelate solution (Hemmilä et al., 1984). A schematic picture of the hypothetical micellar structure into which the fluorescent europium chelate consisting of the europium ion, the β-diketone and the trioctylphosphine oxide molecules is solubilized, is shown in Fig. 2. The high sensitivity and the long lifetime of the europium fluorescence indicate that the quenching effect of water has been almost completely eliminated. When the optimized solution was used for the enhancement of europium fluorescence and a time-resolved fluorometer for measurement, europium was quantitated in a concentration range from 5×10^{-14} to 10^{-7} mol l^{-1} (Fig. 3). Thus at least the same order of sensitivity is obtained as is commonly reported for [125]I (Soini and Kajola, 1983).

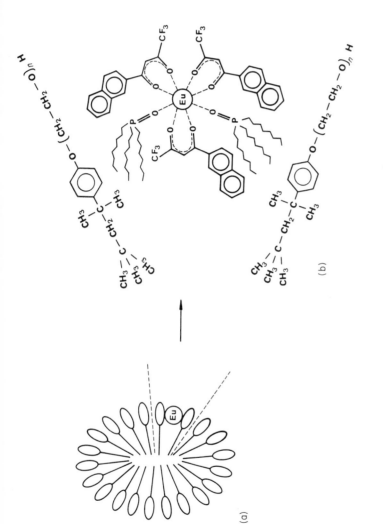

Fig. 2. (a) A micelle consisting of Triton X-100 molecules with an association number of about 140 in which a fluorescent europium chelate is solubilized. (b) A hypothesised form of the europium chelate, consisting of an europium ion, three 2-napthoyltrifluoroacetone and two tri(n-octyl)phosphine oxide molecules as solubilized in between Triton X-100 structures.

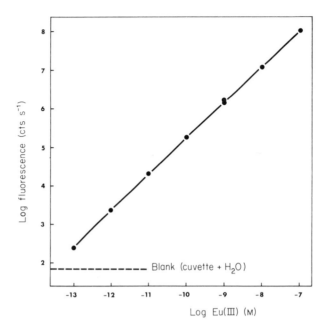

Fig. 3. Dose-response curve for europium. The standards (EuCl₃) were made up in the fluorescence enhancement solution and the fluorescence was measured for 1 s using a time-resolved fluorometer (1230 Fluorometer, LKB–Wallac, 20101 Turku 10, Finland)

4. LINKAGE OF EUROPIUM TO IMMUNOREACTIVE COMPONENTS

In order to use the europium ion as a label in immunoassays, the ion has to be bound strongly to one of the immunoreactive components. Although β-diketones can be used as ligands when measuring europium fluorescence, the stability of the complex is too low for the stated purpose. As it became evidently difficult to combine good absorption and energy transfer properties and strong chelating capacity to the same ligand, an alternative solution had to be considered. If the europium labelling and measurement procedures were separated, the label could be bound efficiently to the immunoreactive component and released from it to form a second highly fluorescent europium chelate which can be quantitated with high sensitivity using time-resolved fluorometry. A strong binding of europium can be accomplished with different polycarboxylic acids, such as EDTA, EGTA, HEDTA and DTPA, which have binding constants for europium in the range 10^{16}–10^{22} l mol^{-1} (Ringbom, 1963). The binding is, however, affected by the environment and consequently, if the conditional constant is calculated for europium under varying conditions such as different pH values (Ringbom, 1963), it becomes evident that europium is readily dissociated from the complex at a low pH. The change in pH from 7–9 to 2–3 decreases the conditional constant drastically and the europium ion is more readily dissociated from the polycarboxylic acid used as chelator. This property is utilized when the pH change is caused by the addition of the enhancement solution containing β-diketone, trioctylphosphine oxide and Triton X-100 at pH 3.2. A highly fluorescent chelate solubilized in the micelles is formed. On the basis of the above principle, polycarboxylic acid based complexones can be used to bind the europium label in a non-fluorescent form to the immunoreactive component. After the immuno-reaction has been completed the europium ion is dissociated from the immunoreactive component into a solution in which the fluorescent chelate arises.

An additional requirement for europium labelling is the introduction of a functional group to molecules such as EDTA which allows conjugation to the immunoreactive component. A useful EDTA derivative, aminophenyl-EDTA, has already been synthesized (Sundberg, *et al.*, 1974) and conjugated to proteins after diazotization. Another alternative is the use of isothiocyana-

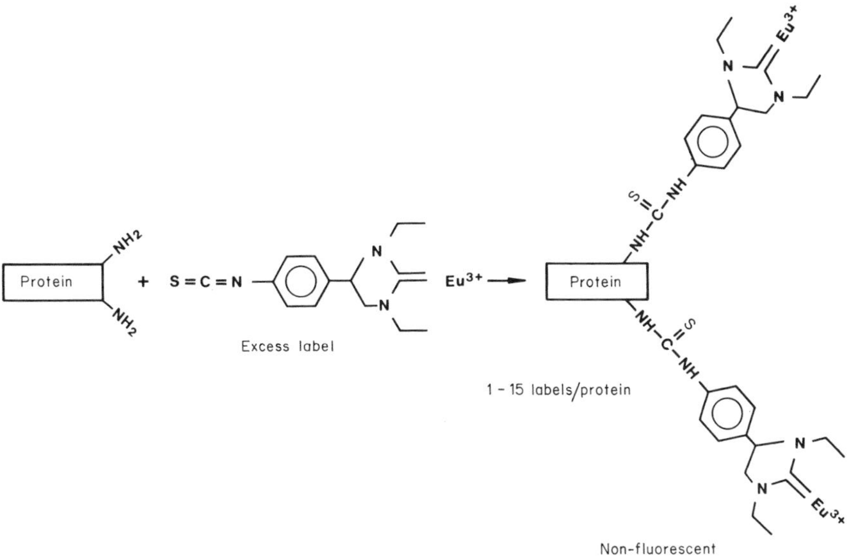

Fig. 4. The principle for labelling of protein with isothiocyanatophenyl-EDTA-Eu. The protein is reacted with a 60-fold molar excess of the label at pH ~ 9.3 overnight at + 4°C. The labelled protein is separated from excess reagent by gelfiltration on a Sepharose 6B column. Conjugation yield is obtained by measuring the europium fluorescence of the labelled protein in comparison with europium standards

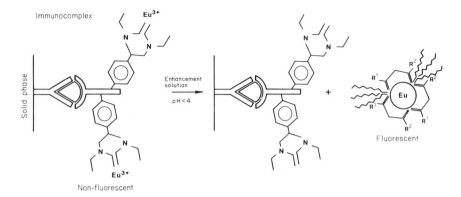

Fig. 5. Principle for the europium release after the immunometric assay has been completed. As a final step before fluorescence measurement an enhancement solution is added consisting of 0.1 M acetone-potassium hydrogen phthalate, pH 3.2, containing 15 μM 2-naphthoyltrifluoroacetate, 50 μM tri(n-octyl)phosphine oxide and 0.1% Triton X-100. The europium ion dissociates from the labelled protein and forms a new fluorescent chelate in solution

tophenyl-EDTA-Eu (Hemillä *et al.*, 1984) which is bound to free amino groups in proteins as shown in Fig. 4. The protein which represents the immunoreactive component is in the procedure actually labelled with a metal ion corresponding to europium in a non-fluorescent form. In an immunometric assay the labelled protein corresponds to the second antibody as shown in Fig. 5. When the immunoreaction has been carried out the enhancement solution is added to dissociate the europium ion from the labelled antibody bound to the antigen on the solid phase. The fluorescent europium chelate is formed in solution and quantitated with time-resolved fluorometry.

5. TIME-RESOLVED IMMUNOMETRIC ASSAYS OF PEPTIDE HORMONES

As it is claimed that the sensitivity of immunometric methods can be significantly increased by the use of non-isotopic labels which display a higher specific activity than that of radioisotopes (Ekins, 1981), it became of interest to test the performance of the time-resolved immunoassay technique based on europium-labelled antibodies for the measurement of human thyrotropin (hTSH) and human chorionic gonadotropin (hCG). Both peptide hormones consist of two subunits (α and β) of which the β-subunit is specific for each of the hormones (Butt, 1983). Since monoclonal antibodies have become available, specific antibodies have been raised against different antigenic sites

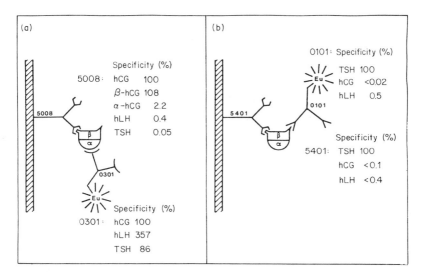

Fig. 6. Immunometric assay principles of hCG and hTSH using europium-labelled monoclonal antibodies. Either one- or two-step assay procedures can be employed. The specificities of the used monoclonals are listed for both assays

on the subunits. These monoclonal antibodies can then be utilized in the immunometric assay of either hTSH or hCG as illustrated in Fig. 6.

In the hCG assay a β-subunit-specific monoclonal antibody is attached to the solid phase and the labelled antibody is raised against the α-subunit of luteotropin (Pettersson *et al.*, 1983). Because of the wide concentration range of hCG generally observed in clinical samples, the assay has been carried out in two steps to avoid the obvious hook effect otherwise observed at high concentrations (>5000 IU l^{-1}). When a simple one-step procedure is performed at least two dilutions have to be tested for a quantitative assessment of the hCG concentration. Scheme 1 provides the detailed assay procedure in the two-step hCG test. The dose–response curve for hCG extends from 1 to 10 000 IU l^{-1} [Fig. 7(a)] with a coefficient of variation below 10% within the whole range. The assay has thus an extraordinarily wide dynamic range with excellent sensitivity. It covers the whole range of hCG values present in different clinical situations with only one dilution.

In the hTSH assay two β-specific monoclonal antibodies directed against different sites were used. The catching antibody was immobilized by physical adsorption into wells of microtitre strips made of polystyrene. The second antibody was labelled with europium (5–10 europium ions per IgG molecule). Because of the low cross-reactivity of the labelled antibody against other peptide hormones (hCG<0.1%, hLH<0.4%) and as no hook effect was

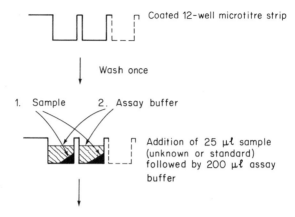

Coated 12-well microtitre strip

Wash once

1. Sample   2. Assay buffer

Addition of 25 μℓ sample
(unknown or standard)
followed by 200 μℓ assay
buffer

Incubate for 1 h at room temperature

Aspirate and wash three times

Tracer

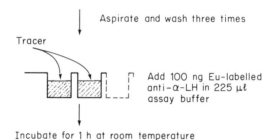

Add 100 ng Eu-labelled
anti-α-LH in 225 μℓ
assay buffer

Incubate for 1 h at room temperature

Aspirate and wash six times

Enhancement solution

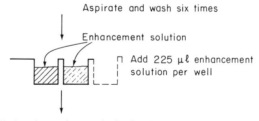

Add 225 μℓ enhancement
solution per well

Shake the strip gently by hand;
after 5 min, measure the fluorescence
for 1 s in a TR fluorometer

Scheme 1. Procedure for the two-step hCG assay

observed within the measuring range, the assay could be carried out in one
step by adding sample or standard and the labelled antibody simultaneously
into the well. A typical dose–response curve for hTSH and a precision profile
for the assay are shown in Fig. 7(b). The sensitivity of the assay is 0.03 μIU
ml^{-1} and the linear range is more than 1000-fold. The precision within the

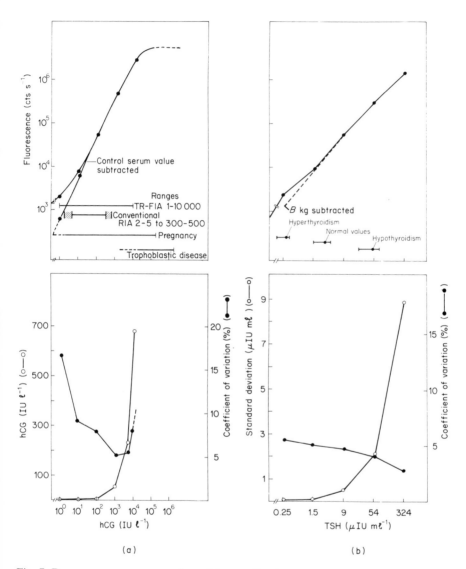

Fig. 7. Dose–response curves and precision profiles for the two-step hCG assay (a) and the one-step hTSH assay (b)

assay range is below 5%. The sensitivity of the assay which goes far below the normal range ($< 1\mu IUml^{-1}$) allows hTSH concentrations to be measured in serum samples of hyperthyroid patients.

The results from the two time-resolved immunofluorometric assays tested as model systems clearly show that very sensitive methods can be developed when antibodies are labelled with europium. Although corresponding assays using the same antibodies have not been set up with radiolabels, it is obvious, e.g. from the sensitivity obtained in the hTSH measurement, that a corresponding value would be difficult to reach with an ordinary ^{125}I label. The high specific activity of the europium label is of great advantage in combination with the immunometric assay principle when an increased sensitivity is required.

6. RAPID ASSAYS OF VIRAL ANTIGENS

For several years sensitive immunoassays have been used for the diagnosis of viral infections (Ling and Overby, 1972). The obvious trend in the development of these assays is to simplify the specimen handling and test procedures so that they can be carried out even in the smallest laboratory and with non-isotopic labels.

Most of the results from the application of immunoassays to the detection of viral antigens have been obtained using time-consuming and laborious indirect assay procedures with several incubation steps. This assay principle has also been used in combination with europium labels and time-resolved fluorescence (Halonen et al., 1983). Recently the test has, however, been simplified by using a direct assay procedure involving only one incubation step which is explained in detail in Scheme 2. The primary capturing monoclonal (Siitari et al., 1983) or polyclonal antibody is coated by physical adsorption on a polystyrene solid phase. The same antibody preparation is used as the second antibody, but labelled with europium. In the assay the occurrence of multiple antigenic determinants (epitopes) is utilized. Although the primary and secondary antibody are the same, both are bound to the

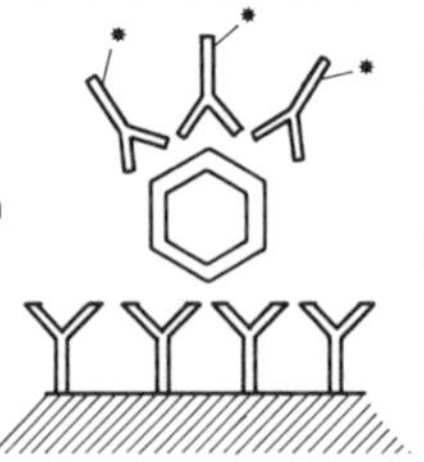

Layer	Immunoreagent		Incubation at 37 °C
	Type	Concentration	
Anti-viral indicator	Eu-chelate-labelled rabbit anti-virus Ig	100 ng per assay	
Specimen	Virus (structural protein)	$0.001-1\,mg\ ml^{-1}$	1 h
Catching antibody	Ig fraction of rabbit anti-virus hyperimmune serum	500 ng per tube	
Solid phase	Polystyrene tube		

Scheme 2. Principle of the direct one-step time-resolved fluoroimmunoassay for the detection of virus antigen

antigen in the one-step assay. Consequently, the assay procedure becomes extremely simple as both the sample or standard and the indicator europium-labelled antibody are added simultaneously. Table 2 shows a comparison of the indirect, direct two-step and direct one-step assay procedures using different amounts of a purified rotavirus reference antigen. The non-specific as well as specific binding is higher in the indirect and the direct one-step assays. The direct two-step assay shows a lower non-specific and specific binding but as their ratio is low the indirect and the direct one-step assay have a higher sensitivity. Obviously more of the labelled antibody is bound to the antigen in the direct one-step assay as compared to the same assay performed by the two-step procedure. The reason for the difference is open for speculation. Polyclonal antibody preparations can apparently be applied to direct one-step immunoassays as well as monoclonal antibodies, provided that the antigen contains multiple identical binding sites. The clinical samples which have been tested according to the direct one-step procedure have shown a good correlation with the indirect measurements using either radioisotopes or time-resolved fluorescence.

Table 2. Comparison of indirect TR-FIA, direct TR-FIA with two incubations and direct TR-FIA with one incubation in the assay of purified rotavirus reference antigen (NCDV)

| | Indirect | | Direct | | | |
| | | | Two incubations | | One incubation | |
NCDV $(ng \, ml^{-1})$	No. counts per second $(\times 10^3)$	(Ratio)	No. counts per second $(\times 10^3)$	(Ratio)	No. counts per second $(\times 10^3)$	(Ratio)
100	53.8	(13)	9.6	(7)	235.0	(55)
10	25.3	(6)	3.1	(2)	28.7	(7)
1	6.9	(2)	1.8	(1.3)	7.9	(1.8)
0	4.1		1.4		4.3	

7. CONCLUSIONS

Immunoassays based on time-resolved fluorescence utilizing europium as the label have led to the following conclusions:

(i) The europium ion is measured as a chelate in solution with high sensitivity.

(ii) The specific activity of the label exceeds that of radioisotopes.
(iii) The europium ion is bound in a non-fluorescent form when used as a label.
(iv) After the immunoreaction is completed the europium ion is dissociated into solution, which facilitates the quantitation based on time-resolved fluorescence.
(v) The high specific activity of the europium label makes it ideal for assays in which high sensitivity is required.
(vi) The label has been applied to immunometric assays of hTSH and hCG using monoclonal antibodies. In both assays a high sensitivity, a wide linear range and an excellent precision have been obtained.
(vii) The label has been used to measure a number of viral antigens using different immunoassay procedures.
(viii) All europium-labelled preparations have already been stable for more than a year when properly handled.
(ix) Europium ions as labels and time-resolved fluorescence as the detection principle are consequently one of the most promising alternatives presently available in the field of non-isotopic immunoassays.

REFERENCES

Butt, W. R. (1983). Gonadotrophins. In *Hormones in Blood*, 3rd edn, Vol. 4 (C. H. Gray and V. H. T. James, eds), Academic Press, London, pp. 137–146.
Crosby, G. A., Whan, R. E., and Alire, R. M. (1961). Intramolecular energy transfer in rare earth chelates; role of triplet state. *J. Chem. Phys.* **34**, 743–748.
Ekins, R. (1981) Merits and disadvantages of different labels and methods of immunoassay. In *Immunoassays for the 80s* (A. Voller, A. Bartlett and D. Bidwell, eds), MTP, Lancaster, pp. 5–16.
Halonen, P., Meurman, O., Lövgren, T., Hemmilä, I. and Soini, E. (1983). Detection of viral antigens by time-resolved fluoroimmunoassay. In *New Developments in Diagnostic Virology* (P. A. Bachmann, ed), Springer-Verlag, Berlin, pp. 133–146.
Hemmilä, I., Dakubu, S., Mukkala, V.-M., Siitari, H. and Lövgren, T. (1984). Europium as a label in time-resolved immunofluorometric assays. *Analyt. Biochem.* **137**, 335–343.
Landon, J. and Kamel, R. S. (1981). Immunoassays employing reactants labelled with a fluorophore. In *Immunoassays for the 80s* (A. Voller, A. Bartlett and D. Bidwell, eds), MTP, Lancaster, pp. 91–112.
Ling, C.M. and Overby, L. R. (1972). Prevalence of hepatitis B virus antigen revealed by direct radioimmune assay with ^{125}I-antibody. *J. Immunol.* **109**, 834–841.
Pettersson, K., Siitari, H., Hemmilä, I., Soini, E., Lövgren, T., Hänninen, V., Tanner, P. and Stenman, U.-H. (1983). Time-resolved fluoroimmunoassay of human choriogonadotropin. *Clin. Chem.*, **29**, 60–64.
Ringbom, A. (1963). *Complexation in Analytical Chemistry*, Wiley–Interscience, New York.

Siitari, H., Hemmilä, I., Soini, E., Lövgren, T. and Koistinen, V. (1983). Detection of hepatitis B surface antigen using time-resolved fluoroimmunoassay. *Nature, Lond.* **301**, 258–260.

Soini, E. and Hemmilä, I. (1979). Fluoroimmunoassay: present status and key problems. *Clin. Chem.* **25**, 353–361.

Soini, E. and Kojola, H. (1983). Time-resolved fluorimeter for lanthanide chelates—a new generation of nonisotopic immunoassays. *Clin. Chem.* **29**, 65–68.

Sundberg, M. W., Meares, C. F., Goodwin, D. A. and Diamanti, C. J. (1974). Selective binding of metal ions to macromolecules using bifunctional analogs of EDTA. *J. Med. Chem.*, **17**, 1304–1307.

Vallarino, L. M., Watsen, B. D., Hindman, D. H. K., Jagodic, V. and Leif, R. C. (1979). Quantum dyes: a new tool for cytology automation. In *Proceedings of the Second International Conference on the Automation of Cancer Cytology and Cell Image Analysis* (N. J. Pressman and J. L. Wied, eds), Tutorials of Cytology, Chicago, Ill., pp. 31–45.

Alternative Immunoassays
Edited by W. P. Collins
© 1985 John Wiley & Sons Ltd

CHAPTER 13

Current concepts and future developments

R.P. EKINS

Department of Molecular Endocrinology,
The Middlesex Hospital Medical School,
Mortimer Street,
London W1N 8AA, UK

1. INTRODUCTION

In this book a number of alternative non-isotopic immunoassay techniques have been reviewed. As is evident from the diversity of the presentations and the amount of research that is being conducted in academic departments and commercial organizations throughout the world, major pressure currently exists to find substitutes for radioisotopic markers for use in the immunoassay field. Aside from what sometimes appears to be an indulgence in methodological novelty for its own sake, a number of more compelling reasons underlie contemporary interest in non-isotopic immunoassay, reflecting a variety of disadvantages attending the use of conventional radioisotopic techniques. Such disadvantages include the supposed biological hazards associated with radioactivity (leading to increasing legal constraints on the use of radioisotopes in certain countries), the cost of radioisotope counting equipment, the limited shelf-life of radioactively labelled reagents, the virtual impossibility of developing isotopically-based non-separation or homogeneous assay methods, the unfamiliarity of laboratory personnel with the use of radioactive techniques, etc.

Some of the reasons offered in support of current interest in alternative immunoassays are nevertheless of dubious validity. For example it is highly unlikely that any non-isotopic assay methodology displaying comparable sensitivity to that of current radioactive methods can be devised which relies on significantly cheaper or more convenient (automatic) instrumentation, especially if the associated data-processing facilities necessary for the maintenance of adequate quality control procedures and other auxiliary equipment are taken into account. Likewise it is equally unlikely that non-separation techniques will ever prove applicable in circumstances in which the very highest assay sensitivity is required. Nevertheless, special problems undoubtedly arise in certain situations (e.g. in Tropical and Third World countries where electrical supplies and instrument maintenance facilities may be unreliable), where a particular logistic advantage of a non-isotopic method may outweigh other disadvantages—such as lack of sensitivity—which it may possess. Bearing in mind the wide variety of circumstances and environments in which immunoassay and other similar binding assay techniques are now employed, it is therefore probable that a number of alternative methodologies will ultimately emerge, each specially suited to the particular circumstances in which it is likely to be used.

Against this background it is perhaps relevant to consider briefly why the radioisotopic techniques have been so widely employed, and established such dominance, in the last 25 years. There are, in my view, two fundamental reasons for this. The first is that radioactively labelled reagents enable the physicochemical reactions on which the protein-binding assay methods are universally based to be monitored even when exceedingly small numbers of molecules are involved, implicitly imparting very high sensitivity to such systems. The second important advantage of radioisotopic labels is the relative invulnerability of the signals which they emit to environmental interference. Radioisotopic disintegration is not affected by physical or chemical factors, and, provided that counting conditions are reasonably well standardized, highly accurate measurements of the radioactive content of individual samples can be made using cheap and easily operable equipment. Moreover, contaminating radioactivity deriving from extraneous sources is not normally present in biological fluids or the reagents customarily used in binding assay procedures, so that measurements are carried out in the absence of high radiation backgrounds. These factors, in conjunction, have provided a secure basis for the development and popularity of the generation of simple, highly sensitive, and relatively rugged radioimmunoassay systems which are in common use at the present time.

In short, though it has long been evident that many different labels may, in principle, be employed to monitor the binding reactions on which the assays rely [indeed the recognition that radioisotopes are not unique in this respect was one important reason underlying my original choice of the general term 'saturation analysis' for the 'competitive' type of binding assay (Ekins, 1960; Barakat and Ekins, 1961; Ekins, 1963)], few markers compare favourably with radioisotopes with regard to their detectability and their invulnerability to environmental factors. In practice, therefore, non-isotopic methods have largely been restricted in their application to the measurement of analytes which exist in biological fluids at relatively high concentrations, and where high assay sensitivity is not a vital requirement.

For these reasons, and because the logistic disadvantage of the radioisotopic methods referred to above do not weigh especially heavily on laboratories in the UK, my own personal interest in non-isotopic assay methodology remained muted for many years. Nevertheless—paradoxically—it has also long been evident in my own laboratory that only by the development of sophisticated non-isotopic techniques would it be possible to penetrate the sensitivity limits characterizing the current generation of radioisotopically based assay methods, and thus to effect a quantum leap in assay methodology comparable with that which took place when the isotopic methods were originally introduced, some 25 years ago.

To put the issue of assay sensitivity into perspective, Fig. 1 portrays the concentration in blood of a very small selection of substances of biological importance, many of which are commonly measured by radioimunoassay. As indicated in this figure, the advent of the radioisotopically-based binding assays for insulin (Yalow and Berson, 1960) and thyroxine (Ekins, 1960) essentially opened up the analyte concentration range extending between 10^{12} and 10^7 molecules per millilitre. Nevertheless, for reasons discussed later in this presentation, analyte concentrations below 10^7 molecules per millilitre lie below the detection limits of current methods. Though it is sometimes argued that it is unnecessary to develop techniques of sufficient sensitivity to penetrate into this region, specific examples occur, even in endocrinology, in which it would be clinically or otherwise useful to increase the sensitivity of present techniques. Moreover in other areas of medicine there is a clear and burgeoning need to measure substances (e.g. tumor, viral and bacterial antigens, etc.) at concentrations considerably lower than 10^7 molecules per millilitre.

The recognition that the development of reliable non-isotopic labels is an essential prerequisite to the penetration of the sensitivity barrier shown in Fig. 1 (rather than a desire to eliminate the relatively minor inconveniences associated with the use of radioisotopes) underlies my own laboratory's interest and involvement in this field. Moreover, the attainment of ultra-high sensitivity also opens the door to many novel immunoassay developments quite aside from the ability to measure substances beyond the sensitivity range of present methods. In this article I therefore propose to examine the question of immunoassay sensitivity and to clarify the reasons why and how non-isotopic techniques form the necessary spring-board from which any future quantum leap in assay methodology must be based. As a necessary preliminary to this examination, I propose to review the fundamental concepts underlying all current binding assay methods.

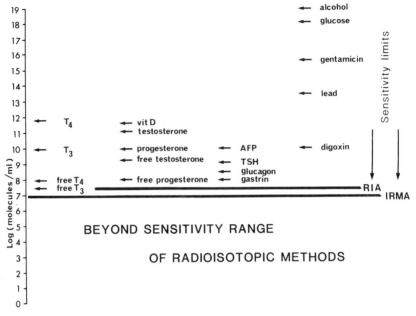

Fig. 1. Approximate concentrations in serum of some typical biologically important substances. The radioisotopically based immunoassay methods made possible the measurement of analyte concentrations falling in the range $10^{12} - 10^7$ molecules per millilitre but do not permit analysis below these levels. [*Note*: The limit of sensitivity shown for IRMA techniques refers to 'non-competitive' systems (see text)]

2. BASIC PRINCIPLES OF BINDING ASSAY METHODS

All analytical techniques rely on observation of the reaction between the analyte and a reagent (Fig. 2), the amount of analyte present being invariably inferred by observing the course, or products, of the reaction. Two basic strategies are available whereby the latter may be achieved: these entail observation of the fate in the system of the analyte (Fig. 3) or alternatively that of the reagent (Fig. 4). Thus in the particular context of protein binding assays (including immunoassays), the analyte concentration may be deduced by observation of the final distribution either of the analyte or of the binding protein (e.g. antibody) between bound and residual (or 'free') compartments following reaction. To facilitate observation of the distribution of analyte or reagent respectively, labelled analyte tracer or labelled reagent tracer may be added to the system (though, in principle, labelling of either of these reactants is not a fundamental prerequisite of the approaches respectively involved). Assuming the binding reagent involved to be an antibody, and the

Analyte + Analytical reagent

↓

Analyte-reagent complex + Residual reagent + Residual analyte

Fig. 2. Fundamental basis of all analytical measurement

label used to be a radioisotope, techniques relying on analyte tracers are generally referred to as 'radioimmunoassay' (RIA); those relying on antibody tracers (i.e. 'labelled reagents') are conventionally described as 'immunoradiometric' assays (IRMA). Analogous terms [e.g. fluoroimmunoassay (FIA); immunofluorometric assay (IFMA)] may be employed to describe techniques relying on other forms of label used to reveal the fate of the analyte or of the reagent in the binding reaction.

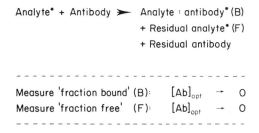

Fig. 3. Analytical method based on 'analyte observation'. Observation of the fate of the analyte following analytical reaction may be facilitated by inclusion of labelled analyte (denoted by an asterisk) in the reaction mixture. Note that the optimal amount of reagent (i.e. antibody) to maximize assay sensitivity approaches zero, irrespective of whether the bound analyte (B) or residual (free) analyte (F) is ultimately 'observed'

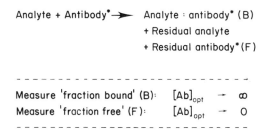

Fig. 4. Analytical method based on 'reagent (i.e. antibody) observation'. In this approach the antibody may be labelled to facilitate its observation. Note that when the bound antibody is measured, the optimal amount of antibody to maximize assay sensitivity approaches infinity

Labelled antibody (IRMA) systems, first introduced by Miles and Hales (1968) and Wide *et al.* (1967) in the late 1960s, were originally claimed to offer greater sensitivity than the corresponding labelled analyte (RIA) methods (Miles and Hales, 1968); however, the validity of this assertion remained controversial for many years. For example in a detailed theoretical analysis Rodbard claimed to demonstrate that labelled antibody techniques were essentially of equal sensitivity to labelled analyte methods (Rodbard and Weiss, 1973); moreover, such differences in the sensitivities obtained in practice using these two analytical approaches could justifiably be attributed primarily to detailed physicochemical differences in the spectrum of antibodies present in the antisera used (and to other similar factors) which prevented any valid and meaningful comparison of the relative performance of the two forms of assay.

In reality, however, the debate relating to the relative sensitivities of RIA and IRMA methods was misplaced, and reflected a misunderstanding of a more fundamental issue. This essentially centres on the differences in optimal assay design which characterize a number of possible alternative immunoassay strategies. In particular it should be noted that the concentration of the analyte in an immunoassay system can be deducted by the measurement (in assays relying on labelled *analyte*) either on the fraction of the labelled analyte which is bound *or* the fraction free. Nevertheless, in both cases it is theoretically demonstrable that the optimal concentration of antibody yielding maximal sensitivity *tends towards zero*. However, the situation is more complicated in assays in which the *antibody* is labelled. In such assays, the optimal concentration of antibody *tends towards infinity* when the bound antibody fraction is measured (assuming negligible non-specific binding of antibody) but *tends towards zero* when the free antibody moiety is observed.

These fundamental differences in assay design are summarized in Fig. 5. This emphasizes that, of the four alternative strategies available, three involve the use of optimal concentrations of antibody tending towards zero, and thus essentially conform to the basic principles of saturation assay. (Such techniques are also frequently referred to as competitive.) In contrast, the fourth strategy permits the use of concentrations of antibody which are high relative to the amounts of analyte present; such systems may be described as reagent excess or non-competitive. Moreover, it is demonstrable that competitive and non-competitive assay systems differ in several important respects—particularly in regard to their specificity characteristics and to the ultimate limitations on their respective sensitivities. In short, when discussing the performance characteristics of different immunoassay strategies, the crucial distinction is *not* between labelled antibody and labelled analyte methods (as represented by IRMA and RIA respectively), but between non-competitive and competitive systems. [*Note:* Rodbard's demonstratioin of equal sensitivity of RIA and IRMA techniques (Rodbard and Weiss,

Labelled Reactant	Measured reaction product	Optimal [Ab]
Analyte	Free	→ 0
Analyte	Bound	→ 0
Antibody	Free	→ 0
Antibody	Bound	→ ∞

Fig. 5. Four alternative immunoassay strategies. Of these, only one (relying on observations of analyte-bound labelled antibody) is 'non-competitive'

1973)—though mathematically correct—was based on the assumption that the *free* antibody fraction is measured, i.e. Rodbard's conclusions related to a competitive labelled antibody methodology.]

It is inappropriate here to discuss in detail the mathematical analyses relating to assay performance underlying these two forms of immunoassay. Nevertheless, some key points emerge from theoretical prediction of the sensitivity limits which arise in competitive and non-competitive assay techniques. In the case of the former, it may be shown that maximal sensitivity attainable with an antibody of affinity constant K is defined by the relative error (δ_R/R) in the measurement of the response variable R (e.g. counts bound) divided by K. However, the error in the measurement of the response is made up of two components: the experimental error component (deriving from pipetting and other manipulations) and the signal measurement error (reflecting, for example, the statistical errors of radioisotope counting).

Assuming, for the sake of simplicity, that the signal measurement error is zero (as would result, in principle, from the use of a radioactive label of infinite specific activity), then the maximal attainable sensitivity is thus given by ϵ/K, where ϵ equals the overall relative error in the response deriving from experimental factors alone (Ekins *et al.*, 1968). For example, if we assume the experimental errors to be of the order of 1%, then the maximal sensitivity achievable using, for example, an antibody with an affinity constant of 10^{12} l mol^{-1} is of the order of 0.01×10^{-12} mol l^{-1} (i.e. 10^{-14} mol l^{-1}). The relationship between maximal sensitivity and antibody affinity is plotted in Fig. 6. However, in practice, signal measurement errors additionally affect sensitivity, and Fig. 6 also illustrates the *actual* sensitivities that are theoretically predictable in an optimized assay system relying on ^{125}I-labelled analyte

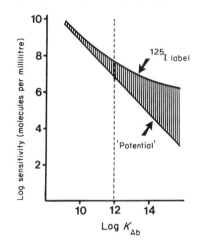
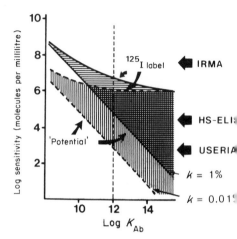
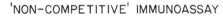

Fig. 6. 'Potential' sensitivities of competitive and non-competitive immunoassay systems as a function of the antibody equilibrium constant (K). The value for ϵ assumed for competitive systems = 0.01 (1%); values for k of 0.01 (1%) (upper curve) and 0.0001 (0.01%) (lower curve) have been assumed for non-competitive systems $\delta n/nsb$ = 0.01 (1%) in both cases.

The '125I' label curves represent the predicted sensitivities attainable assuming labelling of analyte or antibody with ^{125}I (one atom per molecule) and 'reasonable' values for counter efficiency and counting time, etc. Note that for affinity constants below 10^{12} mol^{-1} (the upper limit, in practice, of antibody affinity), the sensitivity loss arising from the use of ^{125}I is small in the case of competitive systems, but may approximate three orders of magnitude in the case of non-competitive techniques. Note also that a non-competitive IRMA may display a sensitivity one to two orders of magnitude greater than a competitive RIA when based on antibody of identical affinity. Arrows indicate typical assay sensitivities reported for non-competitive IRMA, and for analogous enzyme-labelled antibody assays relying on fluorogenic (HS-ELISA (Shalev *et al*, 1980)] and radioactive [USERIA (Harris *et al.*, 1979)] substrates

tracer and using reasonable sample counting times. This diagram thus reveals the extent of a sensitivity gap between the theoretically predicted sensitivity of a competitive assay system relying on ^{125}I-labelled analyte and the maximal sensitivity attainable in a corresponding system in which the signal measurement error *per se* is assumed to be zero. It reveals, *inter alia*, that (unless ϵ is reduced to 0.1% or less) little benefit is potentially derivable in a competitive assay from the use of any alternative label possessing a higher effective specific activity than ^{125}I (which would imply a reduction in the signal measurement error in any specified signal measurement time).

Analogous theoretical considerations apply to non-competitive assay systems and are also summarized in Fig. 6. In an assay system of this kind, the sensitivity obtainable is essentially defined by: (i) the relative error in the estimate of the response (δn/nsb) in the absence of analyte (i.e. by the error in the estimate of the 'non-specifically bound' antibody); (ii) the fractional non-specific binding of antibody (k); and (iii) the equilibrium constant of the antibody (K). In short—making certain reasonable assumptions—the limiting sensitivity of a non-competitive immunoassay (assuming infinite specific activity of the label) is given (Jackson *et al.*, 1983) by $k\delta$n/K(nsb). The maximal attainable sensitivity of both competitive and non-competitive systems is thus inversely related to the affinity constant of the antibody employed, though different proportionality constants [ϵ (i.e. δ_R/R) and $k\delta$n/nsb are applicable in each case. The differences between these constants represents the crucial distinction between the sensitivity potential of these two forms of assay. Thus if we postulate a coefficient of variation in the non-specific binding of antibody of, say, 1%, and a fractional non-specific binding (k) also of 1%, then the maximal sensitivity of a non-competitive immunoassay system is given by $10^{-4}\times(1/K)$, or 10^{-16} mol l^{-1} for an antibody of affinity constant of 10^{12} l mol^{-1} (a value which represents the maximal affinity generally seen in practice).

Figure 6 illustrates two maximal sensitivity curves for non-competitive assays based respectively on the assumption of 1% and 0.01% non-specific binding of labelled antibody. Also shown in Fig. 6 are curves relating assay sensitivity to the antibody affinity constant assuming the antibody used to be labelled with ^{125}I. It is evident that in a non-competitive assay system there exists a large sensitivity loss with respect to that theoretically achievable as a result of the use of ^{125}I as a label. In short, one of the important implications of the analyses summarized in Fig. 6 is that non-competitive systems are capable of yielding assay sensitivities some orders of magnitude greater than competitive assays assuming, *inter alia*, that (i) the fractional non-specific binding of antibody (and other noise-creating effects) can be reduced to approximately 0.1% or less, and (ii) that labels displaying a much higher specific activity than ^{125}I can be identified and utilized.

Though the full sensitivity potential of non-competitive immunoassay systems can only be fully exploited by using non-radioisotopic antibody markers, some advantage nevertheless derives from the adoption of this assay design even when ^{125}I labels are used, as is also revealed in Fig. 6. This figure demonstrates that—depending on the affinity constant of the antibody used (and the assumptions made regarding non-specific binding of antibody, the magnitude of pipetting and other experimental errors, etc.)—it is generally advantageous to employ a non-competitive approach, the sensitivity attainable generally being of the order of 10 times greater (or more) than that of the corresponding competitive design using antibody of identical affinity.

Experimental support for the overall validity of the theoretical predictions summarized in Fig. 6 is provided by: (i) the observation that no radioimmunoassay (or comparable competitive non-isotopic immunoassay system) has yielded a sensitivity significantly higher than 10^{-14} mol l^{-1} (i.e. approximately 10^7 molecules per millilitre); (ii) that (non-competitive) immunoradiometric assays using monoclonal antibodies appear to yield sensitivities up to an order of magnitude greater than corresponding (competitive) radioimmunoassays based on the same antibody; and (iii) the use of labels displaying much higher effective specific activities than radioisotopes (e.g. in consequence of enzyme multiplication of the signal) can, in non-competitive assay designs, yield assay sensitivities extending to below 10^3 molecules per millilitre.

3. OTHER ADVANTAGES OF NON-COMPETITIVE IMMUNOASSAY DESIGNS AND/OR THE USE OF LABELLED ANTIBODIES

Detailed theoretical analysis of the design and sensitivity constraints characterizing non-competitive and competitive immunoassay systems—summarized in the preceding discussion—reveals that sensitivity improvements of many orders of magnitude are *potentially* achievable by the adoption of non-competitive immunoassay strategies. Other advantages which stem particularly from the use of *labelled antibodies per se* (regardless of assay design) derive from (i) their greater stability; (ii) the possibility of using universal labelled reagents (i.e. labelled anti-IgG), and (iii) the avoidance of the problems occasionally involved in the preparation of labelled analyte tracers.

Further advantages deriving from *non-competitive assay designs* include: (i) a shortening of assay incubation times in consequence of the permissible use of relatively high concentrations of antibody; (ii) a reduced dependence upon errors in the pipetting of reagents, and (iii) a reduced dependence upon any minor variations on antibody binding affinity arising from inter sample variability of incubation milieux.

In summary, the use of labelled antibodies in non-competitive immunoassay systems can be predicted to lead to assays of increased speed, sensitivity, specificity (by reliance on two-site assay designs), ruggedness and overall reliability. The main disadvantages of this approach are (i) the need to isolate and label relatively pure antibodies; (ii) the high relative consumption of antibody, and (iii) some increase (in certain protocols) in the number of incubation steps required. Some, at least, of these disadvantages have been obviated by the advent of monoclonal antibody production methods.

In order to exploit fully the advantages of non-competitive assay designs, however, it is clearly necessary to identify labels of higher specific activity than that of commonly used radioisotopes.

4. ALTERNATIVE HIGH SPECIFIC ACTIVITY LABELS

Table 1 summarizes the relative specific activities of some different broad classes of label which have been utilized for immunossay purposes. The conversion of many molecules of substrate by a single enzyme molecule implies an amplification of the specific activity of enzyme-labelled antibody molecules assuming high sensitivity of detection of the reaction product. Examples of high sensitivity non-competitive enzyme-labelled antibody techniques which have exploited this phenomenon are the USERIA technique of Harris *et al.* (1979) and the method of Shalev *et al.* (1980), relying on radioactive and fluorogenic substrates respectively (see Fig. 6). Chemiluminescent labels—in spite of quantum efficiencies generally considerably lower than 100%—are also, in principle, capable of yielding higher specific activities than radioactive isotopes, and hence higher (non-competitive) immunoassay sensitivities. [A recent example of such an assay which may have far-reaching cost–benefit consequences in relation to routine diagnosis of thyroid disease is the high sensitivity measurement of thyroid-stimulating hormone (TSH) which permits the measurement of the sub-normal levels of this hormone which are seen in hyperthyroidism (Woodhead, 1984).]

Table 1. General indication of relative specific activities of commonly used labels

---

Specific activity of ^{125}I

    One detectable event per second per 7.5×10^6 labelled molecules

Specific activity of enzyme label

    Determined by enzyme 'amplification factor' and detectability of reaction product

Specific activity of chemiluminescent label

    One detectable event per labelled molecule

Specfic activity of fluorescent label

    Many detectable events per labelled molecule

Note the low specific activity of ^{125}I. Note also that an enzyme label, by 'amplifying' the number of detectable effects (e.g. using a radioactive substrate) may greatly enhance the effective specific activity of the label and hence the sensitivity of non-competitive assay systems

Fluorescent labels are potentially capable of yielding very high specific activities since each labelled molecule may be induced to yield many photons in response to exposure to a high energy light input. Fluorescent markers also possess a number of other attractive features, including the possibility of confirmatory measurements of the same sample, and the facility they offer for observation of their spatial distribution on a solid surface (thus permitting the ready development of multiple simultaneous immunoassays on the same sample as discussed briefly below). The principal problems associated with fluorescent measurements are the background fluorescence generated by many biological substances, plastics, solvents, etc., and the bleaching effects deriving from continuous exposure of the fluorophore to high intensity light. These disadvantages may be largely obviated by recourse to pulsed-light, time-resolving techniques as discussed in the following section.

5. PULSED-LIGHT, TIME-RESOLUTION FLUORESCENT MEASUREMENT TECHNIQUES

The possibility of employing pulsed-light time-resolution fluorometric immunoassay techniques was first considered in my own laboratory following discussions with J. F. Tait in 1970 who, at this time, proposed the development of a pulsed-laser, time-resolving fluorescent microscope for use in cytological studies. However, because of the high cost of the equipment required and difficulties encountered in funding, studies on the development of such a technique could not be pursued. Subsequently, discussions with Dr E. Soini of LKB–Wallac Oy in the mid–1970s revealed that the rare earth chelate fluorophores offered the possibility of developing pulsed-light, fluorescent techniques employing time-resolving fluorometers of sufficient cheapness to be within the range of small clinical chemistry laboratories. Following development of a prototype instrument by LKB–Wallac, a basic methodology for the attachment of europium chelates to antibodies and a convenient technique for the measurement of the fluorescent signals were developed collaboratively between my own laboratory and LKB–Wallac Oy which have provided the basis for the subsequent development of a range of pulsed light fluoroimmunoassays.

The basic concepts underlying this form of assay (which have already been discussed in some detail in Chapters 7 and 12 of this volume) may be summarized as follows. When a fluorophore is excited by pulsed radiation, fluorescence is emitted following each pulse with an intensity which decreases exponentially with time in a characteristic manner (Ware, 1972). Moreover, as shown in Fig. 7, an electronically gated detection system may be used to accumulate photons emitted over any selected time interval immediately following extinction of the incident light source. Such a system may, in principle, be employed to identify the fluorescent signals emitted by fluorophores characterized by different decay times in a manner which is closely analogous to the approach which has often been employed to resolve mixtures of radioisotopes on the basis of their differing half-lives (Wieder, 1978; Soini and Hemmilä, 1979). However, the simplest and most satisfactory situation clearly exists when a sample contains two fluorophores, one of which

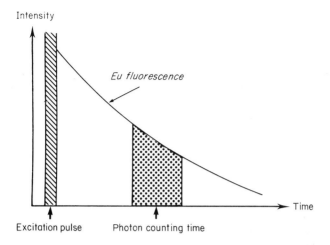

Fig. 7. Time-resolution of fluorescence signal following exposure of fluorophore (e.g. Eu chelate) to short excitation pulse of incident light. Fluorescence photons are 'counted' over any selected counting interval

displays a fluorescent decay time very much longer than the other. In these circumstances it is possible to measure the signal originating from the fluorophore displaying the longer decay time by permitting the more rapidly decaying fluorescence to die away to an insignificant level before commencing photon measurement (see Fig. 8). This simple principle of time resolution can

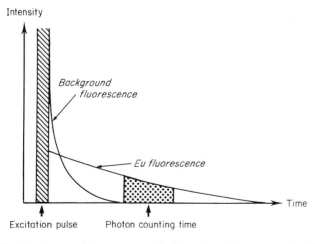

Fig. 8. Short-lived background fluorescence is allowed to fall to an unsignificant level before counting of long-lived fluorescence photons from the fluorophore of interest is allowed to commence

be exploited to reduce or effectively eliminate background fluorescence if this is characterized by a much shorter lifetime than that of the fluorophore of interest, as shown in Fig. 8.

The fluorescence associated with serum proteins and many other common organic substances is characterized by lifetimes of the order of 10 ns (the fluorescence lifetime being defined as the time required for the fluorescence emission to decay to 1/e of its initial intensity following excitation). The lifetimes of some of the fluorophores which are commonly employed in immunochemistry are listed in Table 2. Clearly the simple time resolution method illustrated in Fig. 8 cannot readily be exploited to distinguish between background fluorescence and that characterizing many of the fluorophores, such as FITC or DNS-CL, listed in Table 2; indeed even in the case of NPM (which possesses a lifetime of 100 ns) a significant contribution might be expected from background sources if a substantial proportion of the specific fluorescence deriving from the fluorophore *per se* were to be encompassed within the selected measurement interval of the detection system. In contrast, the fluorescent lanthanide chelates listed in the table form a relatively unique group of fluorophores because of their much extended fluorescence decay times, which are some three to four orders of magnitude longer than those characterizing most background fluorescence. The prolonged decay times of these compounds essentially stem from the delays incurred in the internal transfer processes whereby light energy absorbed by the organic moiety is conveyed to the chelated rare earth atoms which constitute the essential source of the emitted fluorescent photons. Meanwhile, a second useful characteristic of the lanthanide chelates is their large Stokes' shift—that is the difference in the wavelengths of the fluorescent and (optimal) exciting radiations. For example, europium emits fluorescence in a narrow band of wavelengths at around 613 nm; maximal excitation of the chelate occurs using incident light of a wavelength of 340, implying a shift of approx 270 nm. The combination of a large Stokes' shift and an extended fluorescence decay time thus provides the basis for the construction of relatively simple and inexpen-

Table 2. Fluorescence lifetimes of some common fluorophores

	Fluorescence decay time (ns)
Non-specific background	10 ns
Fluorescein isothiocyanate (FITC)	4.5 ns
Dansyl chloride (DNS-Cl)	14 ns
N-3-Pyrene maleimide (NPM)	100 ns
Rare earth chelates	1–1000 μs

sive pulsed light, time-resolving fluorometers capable of yielding exceptionally high signal to noise ratios which are the essential prerequisite of high sensitivity fluorometric measurements.

It is not appropriate to discuss here the problems associated with the labelling of antibody molecules with various lanthanide chelates, and the different techniques available whereby fluorescent signals may subsequently be elicited. For a variety of technical reasons the method developed by Dr Dakubu in my own laboratory (Hemmilä et al., 1984)—which has subsequently provided the basis of the first generation of commercial instruments and assay kits based on these ideas—relies on elution of europium from the chelate-labelled antibody, and measurement of its fluorescence in a solution comprising an appropriately formulated chelating cocktail. Though this clearly entails an additional operation, the elution of europium from antibody into solution occurs in a few seconds or minutes, and necessitates minimal sample manipulation (i.e. the addition of a small volume of the chelating solution to each antibody-containing sample tube). (Amongst other advantages, this procedure reduces inter-sample variation in the measurement of the fluorescent signal using currently available fluorometric equipment.) A number of assays based on this approach have recently been described (e.g. Meurman et al., 1982; Pettersson et al., 1983; Eskola et al., 1983).

However, this development almost certainly represents merely the first stage in the evolution of a range of new immunoassay technologies which I believe will ultimately revolutionize the entire field of microanalysis. Such technologies will almost certainly rely on the measurement of fluorescent molecules localized on a solid surface rather than dispersed in a relatively large fluid volume, thus maximising the signal to noise ratio. For example, one exciting possibility offered by high specific activity, low noise, labels is the development of ambient analyte immunoassays (Ekins, 1982) as exemplified by the two-step free hormone assay techniques originally developed in my laboratory (Ekins and Kurtz, 1979). This form of assay relies on the proposition that introduction of a vanishingly small amount of antibody into an analyte-containing medium results in a fractional occupancy of antibody binding sites which solely reflects the (free) analyte concentration in the medium [regardless of sample volume (Fig. 9) or whether or not the analyte is protein-bound (Fig. 10)]. Fractional occupancy of antibody binding sites is measurable, in principle, in many ways. The procedure adopted in the two-step free hormone assays relies on back titration of residual, unoccupied, antibody-binding sites using appropriately labelled material (e.g. labelled hormone or labelled anti-idiotypic antibody). The use of very high specific activity labels which permit observation of the fractional occupancy of very small numbers of antibody binding sites is clearly obligatory in assays of this kind. Such methodology—which is under active development in my own laboratory—is the basis of the evolution of *in vivo* immunoassay techniques

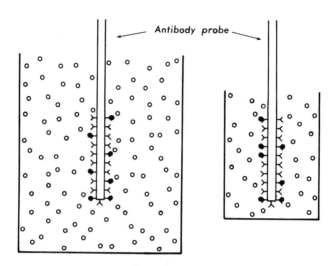

Fig. 9. 'Ambient analyte immunoassay'. The fractional occupancy of antibody sites, given by $[Ab]/[AB_0] = [H] \, K_{Ab}/(1 - [H] \, K_{Ab})$ is determined by the analyte concentration in the medium, $[H]$, and the affinity constant of the antibody, K_{Ab}, and is independent of sample volume. (Antibody-bound analyte molecules represented by black circles).

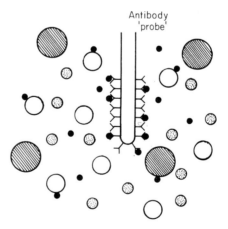

Fig. 10. Principle of 'free hormone' immunoassay. The fractional occupancy of antibody binding sites is governed by the concentration in the medium of hormone molecules (shown in black) which are unattached to molecules of protein (shaded and unshaded circles)

which will permit the measurement of the analyte concentrations existing in particular sites within the body without the necessity for sample removal. This technique also clearly represents the basis of volume-independent forms of dipstick immunoassay which are in the course of development in my own laboratory.

A further possibility offered by fluorescent techniques is that of the simultaneous measurement of many analytes in the same sample by the introduction of a small probe on which is deposited an appropriate array of antibody spots (each of differing specificity) (Fig. 11). Subsequent exposure of the antibody array to a mixture of fluorescent antibodies, followed by scanning of the distribution of fluorescence using a finely focused pulsing light beam, will yield a complete analysis of the analyte composition of the sample. Such an approach could be employed, for example, to obtain a complete hormone profile, or to identify particular viral or bacterial antigens, etc. Obviously the development of a system of this kind cannot be readily accomplished using either radioactive markers or, alternatively, many of the other non-isotopic labels (e.g. chemiluminescent and enzyme labels) whose reactions cannot be spatially resolved in the manner that fluorescent techniques make possible.

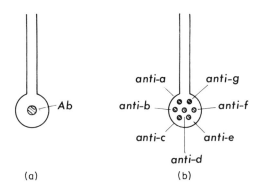

Fig. 11. (a) Simple 'immunometer' (incorporating concept of 'ambient analyte' immunoassay) and (b) 'hormone profile immunometer' permitting simultaneous estimation of a spectrum of different analytes

Looking further into the future, such concepts can be extended to the measurement of ambient analyte concentrations by internal methods of antibody-occupancy recognition by—for example—electronic or optical means. The development of immunoassay methodology along such lines will, *inter alia*, enable the construction of artificial endocrine systems capable of sensing and responding to changing hormonal environments in selected body fluids. Though clearly speculative, there is in my view little doubt that the progressive development of non-isotopic methods of measurement of antibody occupancy will reveal a panorama of microanalytical techniques such as is scarcely visualized at the present time and which will totally transform the immunoassay scene as it exists today.

ACKNOWLEDGEMENTS

Studies in my laboratory relating to the development of the pulsed light, time resolved techniques referred to in this presentation were generously supported by the Sir Jules Thorn Charitable Trust.

REFERENCES

Barakat, R. M. and Ekins, R. P. (1961). Assay of vitamin B_{12} in blood. A simple method. *Lancet ii*, 25–31.

Ekins, R. P. (1960). The estimation of thyroxine in human plasma by an electrophoretic technique. *Clin. Chim. Acta* **5**, 453–459.

Ekins, R. P. (1963). In *Radioaktive Isotope in Klinik und Forschung*, Band V *Vorträge am Gasteiner* (K. Fellinger and R. Hofer, eds). Urban and Schwarzenberg, Munich and Berlin, pp. 211–220.

Ekins, R. P. (1982). Measurement of analyte concentration. UK Patent Application no. 8224600.

Ekins, R. P. and Kurtz, A. B. (1979). Measurement of free ligands. UK Patent Application 7906525.

Ekins, R. P., Newman, B. and O'Riordan, J. L. H. (1968). Theoretical aspects of 'saturation' and radioimmunoassay. In *Radioisotopes in Medicine: in vitro Studies* (R. L. Hayes, F. A. Goswitz and B. E. P. Murphy), Oak Ridge Symposia, Oak Ridge, Tenn., pp. 59–100.

Eskola, J. U., Nevalainen, T. J. and Lovgren, T. N.-E. (1983). Time-resolved fluoroimmunoassay of human pancreatic phospholipase. *Clin. Chem.*, **29**, 1777–1780.

Harris, C. C., Yolken, R. H., Kroken, H. and Hsu, I. C. (1979). Ultrasensitive enzymatic radioimmunoassay: application to detection of cholera toxin and rotavirus. *Proc. Natn. Acad. Sci. U.S.A.* **76**, 5336.

Hemmilä, I., Dakubu, S., Mukkala, V.-M., Siitari, H. and Lovgren, T. (1984). Europium as a label in time-resolved immunofluorometric assays. *Analyt. Biochemistry*, 137, 335–343.

Jackson, T. M., Marshall, N. J. and Ekins, R. P. (1983). Optimisation of immunoradiometric (labelled antibody) assays. In *Immunoassays for Clinical Chemistry* (W. M. Hunter and J. E. T. Corrie, eds), Churchill Livingstone, Edinburgh, pp. 557–575.

Meurman, O. H., Hemmilä, I. A., Lovgren, T. N. and Halonen, P. E. (1982). Time-resolved fluoroimmunoassay: a new test for rubella antibodies. *J. Clin. Microbiol.*, **16**, 920–925.

Miles, L. E. M. and Hales, C. N. (1968). An immunoradiometric assay of insulin. In *Protein and Polypeptide Hormones*, Part I (M. Margoulies, eds), Excerpta Medica, Amsterdam, pp. 61–70.

Pettersson, K., Siitari, H., Hemmilä, I., Soini, E.,, Lovgren, T., Hanninen, V., Tanner, P. and Stenman, U.-H. (1983). Time-resolved fluoroimmunoassay of human choriogonadotropin. *Clin. Chem.*, **29**, 60–64.

Rodbard, D. and Weiss, G. H. (1973). Mathematical theory of immunometric (labelled antibody) assay. *Analyt. Biochem.*, **52**, 10–44.

Shalev, A., Greenberg, G. H. and McAlpine, P. J. (1980). Detection of attograms of antigen by a high sensitivity enzyme-linked immunosorbent assay (HS-ELISA) using a fluorogenic substrate. *J. Immunol. Meth.* **38**, 125–139.

Soini, E. and Hemmilaä, I. (1979). Fluoroimmunoassay: present status and key problems. *Clin. Chem.* **25**, 353–361.

Ware, W. R. (1972). In *Fluorescence Techniques in Cell Biology* (A. A. Thaer and M. Serutz, eds), Springer-Verlag, Berlin, pp. 15–27.

Wide, L., Bennick, H. and Johansson, S. G. O. (1967). Diagnosis of allergy by an in-vitro test for allorgen antibodies. *Lancet ii*, 1105–1107.

Wieder, I. (1978). In *Immunofluorescence and related staining techniques: Proceedings of the 6th International Conference* (W. Knapp, ed.), Elsevier Biomedical Press, Amsterdam, pp. 67–00.

Woodhead, J. S. (1984). In *Monoclonal Antibodies and New Trends in Immunoassays* (Ch. A. Bizollon, ed.), Elsevier Biomedical Press, Amsterdam, pp. 165–174.

Yalow, R. S. and Berson, S. A. (1960). Immunoassay of endogenous plasma insulin in man. *J. Clin. Invest.*, **39**, 1157–1175.

Index

The principal references to facets of immunoassay, and the resultant subdivisions, are listed in alphabetical order.